THE HEALING PO

A comprehensive guide to the
of three products of the beehive: pollen, propolis and
royal jelly.

The Healing Power of Pollen

with propolis and royal jelly

Thorsons Editorial Board

Thorsons Publishing Group

First published 1979
New edition 1989

© Thorsons Editorial Board 1989

British Library Cataloguing in Publication Data

Healing power of pollen. — New ed.
1. Medicine. Natural remedies: Pollen
I. Thorsons Editorial Board
Healing power of pollen
615'.32

ISBN 0-7225-1878-1

*Published by Thorsons Publishers Limited, Wellingborough,
Northamptonshire, NN8 2RQ England*

Printed in Great Britain by Richard Clay Limited,
Bungay, Suffolk
Typeset by MJL Limited, Hitchin, Hertfordshire

1 3 5 7 9 10 8 6 4 2

CONTENTS

ACKNOWLEDGEMENTS

The writing of this book was made possible through the generous help, information, research and time given by those few men and companies who have worked to pioneer pollen, propolis and royal jelly as remedies. All are still engaged in research and development to expand these frontiers of understanding and we take this opportunity of thanking them:

Gösta Carlsson and Åke Asplund of Cernelle, Sweden.
The Horn Family of Ortis, Belgium.
Raymond Matthews of Wassen Developments Ltd, England.
John Peet of Health and Diet Food Co. Ltd, England.
Paul Urban of Melbrosin, Austria.
Mitja Vosnjak, Yugoslavia.

Chapter 1

POLLEN — THE MYSTERIOUS NUTRIENT

Pollen: '*The fine granular or powdery substance produced by and discharged from the anther of a flower, constituting the male element destined for the fertilization of the ovules.*'— Oxford English Dictionary.

Even the dry dictionary definition of pollen conveys some of the mystery and wonder of the substance. But pollen as a food?

Yes, in the same way that wheat germ is now well known to be a valuable and nutritional source of the B vitamins and vitamin E and is so rich in protein that half a cupful contains as much protein as there is in a quarter pound of beef, so pollen researchers are finding more and more precious food substances and micronutrients in the pollen grain.

Extensive medical trials in all parts of the world convince more and more hard-headed and orthodox doctors that the health, virility and vitality of the human body depends not just on the basic food ingredients — proteins, fats, carbohydrates, minerals and vitamins — but also on minute quantities of biologically necessary elements, many of which are found in pollen.

POLLEN THE GIVER OF BALANCE
There are certain parts of the world where people live extraordinarily long lives. Although such areas are continents apart, there is a strong thread linking those groups of people who have a reasonable expectation of being healthy and happy when well past their century.

They are well-balanced in every way, people of deep religious convictions, whether they be Mohammedans as are the Hunzas, Moslems and Russian Orthodox in the Caucasus, and Roman Catholics in Ecuador. They eat little and they eat differently but the result is that they eat a balanced, natural but meagre diet.

The degenerative diseases of western civilization are almost unknown. Hard work, exercise and their diet all contribute to a virtual absence of fat people. They have a real joy of living — singing songs, running races and raising happy children.

Honey, rich with natural pollen, is widely used among such long-lived races and it is most likely that this is a crucial factor in the preservation and maintenance of health. The report of the Lee Foundation for Nutritional Research of Milwaukee stated in 1963 that the composition and nutritional value of the collected pollen is so perfectly balanced that it represents a complete survival food by itself provided that it is extended by roughage and water. The bee-collected content of this diet would need only to be 3 to 4 per cent of the total weight.

Health and happiness are normal states of mankind. Evidence is mounting that, even though the effect may be like a rejuvenation, pollen simply restores balance and normality to many who have lost it for so long that they have forgotten what true health is really like. The extent of the evidence and the remarkable results of pollen supplementation in transforming for the better the lives of countless people is the subject of later chapters. First, a few words about pollen itself.

AMAZING POLLEN

Although the word pollen means, in Latin, pine flour, there is no evidence to suppose that the ancient Romans or Greeks had a special word to describe pollen. Indeed, there is no record of its botanical use until 1523 and it was not in popular usage until the great Swedish botanist Karl Linné, known as Linnaeus, began using it in his descriptions of plants in 1751.

Yet more than 5,000 years ago the Assyrian priests were well aware of the dual sexuality of date palms so, to ensure large crops, they had a ritual of dusting pollen from the male date palms on to the inflorescences of female trees.

So-called primitive peoples knew also of the food value of pollen grains. The early natives of India and the Maoris of New Zealand made cat's tail (Typha) pollen into cakes whilst the Apache and Pueblo Indians used cat's tail (also known as reedmace) and maize pollens in their fertility rites. The Navaho Indians must have been well aware of the balancing properties of pollen because it was part of their 'search for peace'.

Certainly, man must have unwittingly taken a lot of pollen in honey. It is only recently that honey has been strained so that much of the pollen is removed. Regrettably, many of the cheap honeys are not only finely filtered but also heat treated so that the natural and vital enzymes are destroyed, turning honey from a healthy food into just another calorie-laden sweetener.

The pollen grain has around it two protective and durable coats. The outer waxy exine is made of sporopollen which is able to resist most acids and temperatures as high as 300°C. Beneath this is the fragile inner wall, the intine, which surrounds and protects the nuclei and the reserves of starch and oil.

The pollen grain is physically so indestructible that identifiable grains are found in the earliest geological strata from the time when, millions of years ago, plants first bore pollen grains.

Even the largest pollen grains are so minute that more than 14,000 of them would be needed to weigh a single gram or over 400,000 grains to one ounce. Small pollen grains such as that of the spruce tree weigh only one-twentieth of this so that an ounce would require the staggering total of more than eight million pollen grains!

An idea of the vast numbers of pollen grains which must cover the earth since the first possible traces 300 million years ago can be gained from the fact that the spruce forests of southern Sweden alone deposit 75,000 tons of pollen a year upon the surrounding countryside. This is equivalent to 10-followed-by-twenty-noughts grains of pollen!

There are wide variations in the size of a pollen grain ranging from, at the smallest end for a plant like Myosotis, two microns across. That means that almost 13,000 would be required to be laid end to end to represent just one inch. One of the largest pollen grains, on the other hand, is that of Eelgrass. This measures no less than 2,550 microns long by 3.3 microns wide. It would take only ten of these to make up our inch.

The number of grains produced by a plant can be equally extreme ranging from *Araucaria* (a genus of conifers) which has a thousand million grains from a single male cone, to one maple floret which has but eight thousand.

POLLINATION

The act of transference of pollen from the anther to the stigma is called pollination, but the actual process of fertilization can take much longer. In some species the process takes less than a day; in others, such as *Agathis*, a year; and in Juniper, fifteen months.

Sometimes, plants are able to pollinate themselves and when pollen is transferred from the anthers of one flower to the stigma of another of the same species it is called cross-pollination which, like sexual reproduction in animals, keeps alive the vitality of the species. The pollen may be transferred, as in the case of the buttercup, by the action of insects or it may be carried on currents of air. The wind-pollinated plants tend to have far more grains of pollen than do those that are insect-pollinated and it is when these wind-pollinated plants are shedding their pollen that most attacks of hay fever occur.

THE COMPOSITION OF POLLEN

Pollen is so complex that the time is not yet in sight when we will have a precise analysis of it. Indeed, there are certain to be differences between various plants, some of which have already been established. The two main analyses were done by the Lee Foundation and by the Swedes, Nielsen, Grömmer and Lundén in 1955.

There was also an important analysis by Vivino and Palmer of the University of Minnesota in 1944 but they lacked some of the sophisticated pieces of apparatus available to the more modern researchers.

Table 1 in the Appendix shows the basic composition of pollen, and Table 2 lists the amino acids present in three different pollens. Amino acids are the constituents of proteins — the muscle builders of our bodies. Table 3 indicates the actual quantities of some of the more important amino acids present in four pollens one of which is sampled over successive years to show that there are seasonal variations but that these would not appear to be very large.

Table 4 shows that important quantities of vitamins are also to be found in pollen. Table 5 gives an analysis of the fatty acids in pollen.

In addition to the vitamins shown in the table other work has demonstrated the presence of pro-vitamin A, vitamin D, vitamin E, vitamin B1 (thiamine), choline, vitamin C (ascorbic acid), vitamin K and rutin.

Many authorities believe that it is much more important to have a balanced and widely spread supplementation of vitamins than to take large quantities of a single one, except when there is a special need. Pollen clearly provides a good fundamental vitamin supplementation when used in addition to a normal healthy diet.

The minerals identified in pollen include sodium, potassium, magnesium, calcium, aluminium, iron, copper, zinc, manganese, lead, silicon, phosphorus, chlorine and sulphur. Enzymes already discovered in pollen include amylase, catalase, cozymase, cytochrome systems, diaphorase, diastase, lactic dehydrogenase, pectase, phosphatase, saccharase, and succinic dehydrogenase.

Chapter 2

COLDS AND FLU

'The bee is more honoured than other animals, not because she labours, but because she labours for others.' — St John Chrysostom, in about the year 383.

One sometimes wonders whether the only people who have not got a useful remedy for colds are those who work at the British Government's Cold Research Centre on Salisbury Plain!

Professor Osmanagic has, among others, shown how effective is another bee-gathered product, the resin called propolis, in preventing and treating influenza and other infections, and all producers of pollen products are able to show me sheaves of unsolicited letters from those who have either prevented colds during an epidemic or been cured of their infections in record time through taking their daily pollen.

The scientist rightly requires clinical trials and it must be admitted at once that there is plenty of scope for more work and more trials on pollen for colds and influenza. But the tests that have been carried out so far are really very exciting in their excellent results.

No one is claiming a miraculous freedom from colds and influenza or a complete cure within hours. The most that the average sufferer desires is to be well enough to continue work and not be a burden to himself and to others as he suffers. A wave of flu enveloped Sweden between February and May 1967, which is when a heavy industrial company in Sweden, worried about absence through illness, decided to experiment with *Fluaxin*, a mixture of aspirin and pollen extract produced by Cernelle containing in each tablet 110 milligrams of pollen extract and 100 milligrams of aspirin.

By the end of May, 510 employees had been given a total of 908 packets containing 5,448 *Fluaxin* tablets. Of these, only 9 succumbed to influenza, 6 reported sick after one packet of tablets, 2 after two packets and 1 after five packets. The conclusion of Doctor Klapsche, who was controlling the trial, was that he had received the impression that *Fluaxin* was a thoroughly useful agent in influenza prevention and therapy. The intake of the tablets enabled 98 per cent of their employees who suffered from influenza to continue working in heavy industry, avoiding the necessity of them taking time off because of sickness, therefore the results appear to be quite remarkable. The aspirin would be included for its beneficial effects on headache and temperature. It certainly has no effect on the actual influenza.

In April 1976 the two Yugoslavs Filipic and Likar, of The Medical Faculty of the Institute of Microbiology in Ljubljana, published a paper called *Inhibitory Effect of Propolis and Royal Jelly on some Viruses* in which they began:

'Propolis, royal jelly, pollen and honey are natural products of bees. They have a variety of effects: biological, physiological and antimicrobial. For medicine the anti-microbial effect is of some interest. It is known from clinical experiences that they are active against bacteria, yeasts and fungi. In our experiments we made an attempt to determine their activity against viruses pathogenic for man.'

They went on to use influenza virus A2 and Vaccinia virus which is the one responsible for smallpox. They discovered that the multiplication of the influenza virus was much reduced by a mixture of propolis and royal jelly and that the inclusion of royal jelly was important to a successful result. But in the case of the smallpox virus the propolis alone was enough and the royal jelly had no added effect.

Another very important finding was that the royal jelly, to be effective, had to be natural and not chemically treated or dried. Many of us would have expected this to be so through the knowledge that there are many enzymes present which would be destroyed after such treatment. We have investigated the production methods of two of the main producers of royal jelly health products which are Ortis of Belgium and Melbrosin in Austria: they both go to tremendous lengths to ensure that the royal jelly that they use is gathered from the young larvae when it is most potent, and it is stored under ideal conditions before incorporation into the products.

COMPLEX OF SUBSTANCES

Filipic and Likar believe it is possible that there is not only one active substance but a whole complex of substances which exert their full physiological and anti-viral effects only when in a proper mixture. When this happens there is an inhibition or a prevention of infection.

This sounds a warning against those scientists who, as soon as they discover a beneficial effect, seek to isolate the active principle and make a tablet out of it. We are coming to realize more and more that even the apparently useless part of food, for example the bran part of wheat, can be beneficial to mankind who in the course of evolution has grown up with the whole of nature and not just refined and isolated parts of it.

The oft-repeated argument that man is nothing but a mixture of chemicals anyway so why worry about adding a few more is shallow and does not stand close examination. Yes, of course, we are a mixture of chemicals, but those chemicals are produced in forms which constitute the basic building blocks of nature. We are far better off if we feed and treat our bodies with natural substances that are harmoniously balanced with nature as these are far less likely to produce undesirable side-effects.

Of course, one must not decry the magnificent advances in medicine and in the use of quite artificial materials to control disease, but in fifty years' time I believe that very many of these 'cures' will be looked upon as useful stop-gaps in man's medical progress and that many more natural substances will have replaced most of the synthetic pharmaceuticals.

The success of the experiments on heavy industry workers led to further trials to establish the effectiveness of the Cernelle pollen preparations on upper respiratory infections in general. Dr John Glømme, of the University of Oslo, brought together the work of several scientists over a period of six years to try and see exactly what effects the Cernelle pollen tablets have on such diseases. He found that this was very difficult because all the workers had adopted rather different approaches and anyway it is not at all easy to prove that you would have had a cold if you had not taken a certain preventive treatment! But he concluded that statistically there was, overall, a reduction in the amount of sick leave and in visits to the doctor for these diseases, with less pronounced symptoms and a shorter duration of illness, as well as a general increase in the feeling of well-being which made the taking of the pollen thoroughly worthwhile.

He believed that all these results could be put down to the general strengthening effect of taking pollen.

Finally, if you have a cold, or indeed any infection or wound, there are great drains on the body's reserves of vitamin C. Indeed, the smoking of a single cigarette is said to use up 30 mg of vitamin C which is half as much as many authorities believe people need in a single day. So, if you smoke you may well need extra vitamin C and you certainly will if you have a cold or other infection or injury.

It is always a good idea to take one gram of vitamin C every two or three hours at the first sign of a cold, reducing the dose to about two or three grams a day if the cold persists more than two or three days. We are not at a sufficiently advanced state of knowledge to be able to say that man should consume many grams of extra vitamin C every day although many have done so without apparent ill-effect.

So, take a course of pollen, preferably, but not necessarily, with royal jelly every winter and the chances are that you will avoid serious colds and respiratory infections even if those around you are suffering from the seasonal sniffles.

Chapter 3

HAY FEVER, ASTHMA, ALLERGIES AND THE PERSORPTION PHENOMENON

'Men are less sensitive to good than to ill.' — Livy 10 B.C.

Those who suffer from hay fever and other allergies such as eczema and asthma are often very worried about the idea of actually consuming pollen. They believe that they are simply asking for trouble!

Experience is quite different. Although a very small percentage of people (estimates vary from 1 in 2000 to about 5 per cent) find that propolis brings them up in a slight rash, pollen is not known to have any such effect. The reason for this is often given that hay fever is caused by wind-borne pollens while most pollen products are made from bee-gathered pollen; but this does not explain the desensitization effect of pollen which often, but not always, has a very beneficial effect upon sufferers from hay fever.

The distinguished natural doctor, Dr Gordon Latto, talked about his results in his beautiful and organically cultivated garden just outside Reading one fine summer's day when the bees were busy supplying his ten home-made hives with precious honey.

He took us to his cellar where he stores the honey and showed us many jars which all had one unusual factor in common. There was a thick messy looking scum on top of each jar. This was where the pollen which had not been filtered away had risen to the top. He gives his hay fever patients a little bit on the end of a spoon every week for about six weeks before the beginning of the hay fever season and the usual result is that they have reduced attacks in the first year and are often completely free from hay fever by the second year.

It is certainly worth trying pollen if you suffer from eczema, asthma, hay fever or a similar allergy, because there are very many letters from former sufferers in the files of the suppliers of pollen testifying to successful treatment often after many years of suffering. On the other hand it must be realized that, as Dr Richard Mackarness discovered, there are many unsuspected allergenic substances all around us, including many common foods, and often a cure will only be achieved by undertaking a short fast and then adding one item only of food to your diet every three days until you discover which have a harmful effect. This is best done under the supervision of a sympathetic practitioner who will make sure that you do not suffer any nutritional deficiencies.

A very interesting research project was carried out in Sweden in 1960 and reported on in *Grana Palynologica* Volume 2 in that year by Einar Helander who had treated, in the allergy department at Gothenburg, some 2,072 patients with pollen allergies. He chose 25 patients who were allergic to pollen but otherwise healthy and found that although they were extremely allergic when given a skin test made up of the ground tablets, when taken by mouth, even in a large dosage, such small amounts of pollen antigen were absorbed that he recommended a trial for the product in the desensitization of hay fever sufferers. Let us hope that this important trial is not too long delayed.

THE PERSORPTION PHENOMENON
New research has centred on the remarkable observations that even a person who is sensitive to an allergenic pollen does not necessarily exhibit the symptoms of the allergy when taking pollen tablets. It is now thought to be because some of the pollen particles pass directly from the stomach into the blood-stream. Such passage is called persorption. This is far more rapid than the normal processes of digestion and indeed pollen can be observed in the blood and urine and spinal fluids only two hours after the pollen has been eaten.

Limskens and Jorde found in 1974 that, when 150 grams of pure rye pollen were eaten, between six and ten thousand grains were persorbed into the blood-stream. Upon examination the tough exine or outer coat of the pollen was found to be partially destroyed, a process that continues with time.

Although much more study is needed and indeed is being undertaken on this remarkable phenomenon, it is already believed that taking whole pollen tablets for some six months before the hay fever season may bring about immunity because of the persorption effect. The time may come when pollen tablets are made with different mixtures of pollens suitable for sufferers from different forms of hay fever.

Chapter 4

POLLEN FOR THE PROSTATE, FOR RHEUMATISM AND ARTHRITIS

'Old vessels must leak.' — Torriano A.D. 1666

Alin Caillas reports that in France 30 per cent of all men over the age of 50 suffer from enlargement of the prostate gland. This little walnut-sized gland lies around the exit tube from the male bladder, and enlargement is certainly very inconvenient, causing an excessive frequency of passing of water, especially at night. Even worse is the fact that the sufferer is unable to entirely empty his bladder; altogether an unsatisfactory state of affairs. This is often combined with an inability to pass water which can only be relieved by the introduction of a tube into the bladder. The condition can often be entirely controlled by good treatment without the need for an operation, and indeed the operation when carried out is nearly always very successful.

It is good to know that pollen has helped quite a few sufferers from enlarged prostate but it would be exaggerating to suggest that it is by any means always successful. However, reports are sufficiently encouraging to make it a worthwhile treatment especially in the early stages. The use of pollen is far better established in the case of prostatitis.

PROSTATITIS

Prostatitis is an inflammation of the prostate gland and is often accompanied by pain together with symptoms quite similar to those of an enlarged prostate. Dr Ask-Upmark of Uppsala reported in 1967 the treatment of 12 cases with Cernelle pollen at a dosage of five to six tablets a day taken first thing in the morning. Only

2 cases out of 12 had a negative result and the improvements were striking in the 10 successful patients both from the sufferer's point of view and upon careful clinical examination.

The failure in the first case was due to another medical complication. The second was a middle-aged Norwegian shipowner who was in the habit of wading in the icy cold Norwegian rivers with the water well above his knees in order to indulge in his sport of salmon fishing. His refusal to alter this habit was, in the opinion of Dr Ask-Upmark, surely likely to accelerate his prostatitis and accordingly the treatment was discarded.

A German-Swedish investigation by a team of distinguished urologists, Alken, Jönsson and Röhl, reported their investigations into 172 cases of prostatitis at about the same time. They found that the pollen preparation produced relief in no less than 44 per cent of cases, a figure which they found very satisfactory.

One of the patients in the first group was a striking example of the long-term effects of pollen consumption in that he had suffered from prostatitis between the ages of 50 and 55 when he began taking *Cernilton*. The doctors, pronouncing a cure, have tried in vain to persuade the patient to give up the pollen treatment because he remembered a period of two weeks near the beginning of the administration of pollen when, being abroad, he had forgotten to take his tablets and suffered a relapse of the disease. He was accordingly scared of giving up his medication and has so far seen no ill-effects after nine years consumption of pollen.

Another trial by the Professor of the Urological Clinic of Magdeburg, Professor Heise, used the pollen for three years in a trial of nine patients who not only had difficulty with passing water but also found cohabitation was difficult and had bacterially positive emissions.

Suicide had been attempted by two of the patients and four others were very depressed. A three-year treatment with pollen showed that in all nine cases the bacteria were absent after a course of one tablet taken three times daily and that all the patients exhibited a considerable improvement both mentally and physically, no longer had difficulties with their marital relationships and the passing of water became normal. Professor Heise concluded that it would be a commendable advance if treatment with this pollen preparation were to become incorporated into recommended therapeutic practice.

RHEUMATISM AND ARTHRITIS

One producer of pollen products, Pollen-B, has found that sufferers from rheumatism and arthritis have often been amazingly improved when on a course of their preparation.

They have been so much influenced by the very large number of letters written to them claiming good results that they are carrying out a long-term medical trial in order to discover the precise action of pollen upon these crippling disabilities.

These two letters are typical of many:

E.T., London SE9

I had read about your Pollen-B tablets earlier this year and bought a three month supply in July because for some weeks I had been suffering with severe arthritis in the knee and in the arm.

I have now finished the three months course and to my delight I feel no pain in these joints and at this time of year (October) it usually gets worse especially as I had it during the summer.

A.J.P. Gerards Cross

I feel I should write to you as a result of following the recommendation of a friend to try a course of Pollen-B. At my age (75) with a lengthy history of treatment for fairly severe arthritis, necessitating the taking of numerous sophisticated drugs in some quantity and at a somewhat irksome frequency.

To my pleasant surprise, as a result of taking Pollen-B, not only have I felt increasingly better in myself but, what is more revealing, I have been able to cut down on the taking of certain drugs previously essential for maintaining my mobility.

Therefore I feel it only right that I should express my personal appreciation of Pollen-B if only to convey to others the possibility that this food supplement could be beneficial and it is at least worth a trial course.

The changes to bones in severe arthritis are not reversible but it does seem that even severe cases have derived some benefit from the taking of pollen. It is certainly a good idea, if you suffer from one of these conditions, to give a pollen a three months trial — in any case you will feel much better! At the same time, there are other useful supplements you can take, such as evening primrose oil with marine (fish) oils, and selenium with vitamins A, C and E.

Chapter 5

HAIR AND SKIN, AND RADIATION SICKNESS

'There is no need to call a hairdresser for your head. A sponge, Phoebus, would do the business better.' — Martial A.D.90

Nettle juice, jojoba oil, mixed spinach and lettuce juice consumed for six months are all reputed to restore hair. Indeed, there is evidence that all these have worked. To this list we must certainly add pollen. There have been many reports, especially from those who have lost hair later on in life, of a new strong growth of hair appearing after the taking of a long course of pollen tablets for some other reason.

It could well be that the reason for the beneficial effect of pollen on hair growth and on arresting the loss of hair is because the pollen grain is rich in the amino acid, cystine. The composition of hair includes 17 per cent of cystine so that if there is a deficiency of this important amino acid in the diet the growth of the hair is certain to be affected. Baldness comes from many different causes and there is an important hereditary factor which is also involved. So pollen will not work for everyone, but it is good to know that an improvement in hair colour and growth of new hair can be a welcome additional bonus to those who take pollen regularly.

POLLEN FOR THE SKIN

The beneficial effects of pollen in some cases of allergy have already been mentioned in Chapter 3. Dr Lars-Erik Essen found that the application of pollen products to the skin were of value in his cosmetic and dermatological work. He found that there was a suppressive effect in facial acne and that pollen preparations facilitated the healing and treatment of burns.

It is already well-known that honey itself provides a very good treatment for burns and wounds and has even been used in hospitals for that purpose. It could be that the pollen and propolis content of the honey plays a part in the healing process and that all these ingredients work together in harmony.

If you are using pollen on the skin it is certainly a good idea to also take it by mouth because undoubtedly pollen increases the resistance and builds up a higher threshold against fatigue, permitting the human organism to heal itself under the most favourable circumstances.

RADIATION SICKNESS

Professor Osmanagic and his colleagues carried out some important trials with Melbrosin pollen capsules at the University Radiological Institute of Sarajevo during 1973.

They had been much concerned because, even with the most up-to-date techniques, patients undergoing X-ray therapy quite often showed adverse reactions because of the effect of the X-rays on the blood. There are also digestive troubles which occur when radiation is carried out on a large surface of the abdominal region involving loss of appetite and sickness. Sometimes, indeed, the discomfort was so great that the treatment had to be interrupted because the general condition of the patient was threatened. It seems that the X-rays break down the body's proteins producing histamine with resultant allergic effects.

The Melbrosin product which was used contained royal jelly and fermented pollen and was chosen because it was felt that the very wide content of naturally occurring supplementary substances should have a broad spectrum of activity. The first positive effect they found was that the liver was greatly improved in function with a four-fold increase in the formation of glycogen.

The product was tested on 16 women patients who all had radiation sickness of various intensity. The blood and the liver were analysed so that there was laboratory confirmation that the patients suffered from classical radiation sickness. The most frequent troubles experienced by the patients were tiredness, fainting, loss of weight, loss of potency, nausea and vomiting. Also, anaemia was present in 12 of the patients and liver damage in almost all of them. It was found that the liver analysis became normal in the case of 10 patients even though they carried on with the radiation treatment; 9 women had an improvement of the red blood picture and 9 of the white blood.

The improvement in the general condition of these women and the reduction of their subjective trouble was even more significant. They were lessened in all cases and disappeared entirely in most of the patients.

Professor Osmanagic then checked his findings by taking two further groups, one of 29 patients who took a Melbrosin capsule twice a day, in the morning and the evening, for forty days, and another group of 30 patients in the same condition who were given a harmless placebo made to look like the Melbrosin capsules, for the same period. A third group of 31 patients with the same symptoms of radiation sickness were given no medication at all.

All but 2 of the patients who had been treated with the placebo preparation showed a general deterioration in their state of health during further radiation treatment as did all the untreated patients. Of the 29 patients taking the pollen and the royal jelly preparation, 2 reported only a slight improvement, 13 a good result and 14 a very good effect resulting in the virtual elimination of all the unpleasant effects of radiation.

Chapter 6

WOMEN'S PROBLEMS

'Health is beauty, and the most perfect health is the most perfect beauty.' — Shenstone 1764

Never before has it been so challenging or so rewarding to be a woman. Whether your role is that of an elegant efficient business woman, a loving wife and mother, a busy factory or shop worker, never before has there been such a need for you to be on top of things with radiant health, abundant energy and strong self-confidence to carry you safely through an exacting day.

Yet the very nature and physiology of a woman creates extra pressures and difficulties that do not exist for most men. Even if a woman goes out to work, if she has a family and a house to run she is expected to do all that as well. For more than thirty years of her life she has menstrual periods which can be uncomfortable, occasionally cause psychological disturbances and, for one in ten, cause some anaemia.

To cap it all, many women have a difficult menopause as the whole rhythm of their life alters in middle age. Yet through all this and through the strains of life womanhood is expected to portray charm, femininity and beauty.

Is it then a coincidence that the pollen from the flowers which are so often given as symbols of love and as a tribute to femininity today helps so many women to overcome, in a natural way, many of those special problems, which are so often just taken for granted as an inevitable fate.

Important clinical tests have been made on a pollen product that has been specially designed for women, *Melbrosia PLD*

(Florapoll), capsules containing a blend of specially selected pollens and royal jelly.

MENSTRUAL PROBLEMS

Dr Bogdan Tekavcic, the head of Ljubljana Centre for Gynaecology, conducted tests on two groups, each of 30 girls between the ages of 18 and 22. The first group were underweight, had irregular menstruation and very painful periods. The second group had only the painful periods and did not have any other menstrual problems.

Half the girls in each group took a placebo capsule containing no active ingredients for two consecutive months. The remaining girls took one capsule a day of *Melbrosia PLD* for two months.

The results were striking. More than three-quarters of the underweight girls gained between 1 and 3 kg (2 and 6½ lb) whereas only a quarter of the control group gained weight.

In both groups the menstrual pains failed to either disappear entirely or be considerably diminished in only two girls out of each of the groups taking *Melbrosia PLD,* whereas only 6 out of the 30 girls taking the placebo had any improvement at all. Furthermore the improvement for the girls taking the pollen and royal jelly was usually evident after the first month — and all this with no untoward side-effects at all!

HELPING THE 'CHANGE'

Dr Tekavcic selected 74 women aged between 40 and 55 years who, although still menstruating, were showing definite symptoms of the change of life. Of these, 38 took one daily capsule of *Melbrosia PLD* on an empty stomach for two consecutive months and the remaining 36 took a similar-looking placebo. This is so often a time of life when women put on weight, yet of the 38 cases taking the pollen 20 lost weight and only 7 increased in weight. In the placebo group only 4 lost any weight. This was a most helpful and unexpected result which had not been anticipated.

The presence of unpleasant side-effects in these women was graduated on a scale numerically and this was called the Climacteric Index. After they had taken the course of capsules the women were carefully examined against the same scale and the improvements or lack of them were recorded.

Out of 38 cases taking the capsules 35 recorded a considerable reduction in the C.I. A wonderful result! 17 of the 38 had been recorded as suffering from particularly severe menopausal problems of an index figure of between 30 and 36. After treatment 34 cases out of 38 had a C.I below 19 indicating a minimal degree of symptoms.

In 14 cases the C.I. even fell below 10 which means that the change of life was then without any troubles at all.

THE OLDER WOMAN
Doctor Tekavcic, having had a successful experience with women who were undergoing their change, then turned to the group who had not menstruated for at least a year but still suffered from symptoms strong enough for them to seek medical advice.

He chose a similar number of women aged between 40 and 65 years and divided them into a placebo group of 38 cases and a group treated with *Melbrosia PLD* of 37 cases.

Of those taking treatment 18 lost weight and of the untreated group only 7 recorded a weight reduction. When he came to the Climacteric Index, the C.I. was reduced in 34 out of 38 cases in the group taking the treatment whilst only 10 had an improvement in the control group.

HELPS THE BRAIN TOO!
Both the girls who were students and the women who were at the clinic because of their problems of middle age made specific mention to their medical adviser that there were two additional effects which, they felt, must be mentioned. First of all they had a great increase in their powers of mental concentration and, secondly, there was an obvious influence for the better on their normal sexual enjoyment which had previously tended to be inhibited because of their personal problems.

The doctor concluded that although he would have expected an improvement because of the psychological effect of any capsule taken by women at the time of the change or girls suffering

from painful periods, the differences between the control groups
and the groups taking the *Melbrosia PLD* capsule were very striking and statistically significant, proving to his satisfaction that
the product had an extremely beneficial effect.

FURTHER PROOF

The head of the gynaecological department at the University of
Sarajevo is the distinguished Professor Doctor Izet Osmanagic,
mentioned in Chapter 5. During the course of his work he has
gained much experience in many parts of the world in important
hospitals and it is this professor who decided to see whether the
results of Doctor Tekavcic could be confirmed.

He was particularly interested to see whether many problems
of the 'change' such as hot flushes, perspiration, headaches and
palpitations could be helped. He carried out his trials over a six
month period.

The scale of the Climacteric Index was between 1 and 36 and
the values of both his groups lay between 12 and 26. Five of his
patients were aged between 30 and 40, 28 between 40 and 50
and 7 between 50 and 60. Their complaints were classified so
that to have no complaints was scored as nought; slight complaints
were scored as 1; distinctly recognizable complaints 2; complaints
of a serious nature 3. He evaluated a 25 per cent reduction in
complaints as slightly successful, a 50 per cent reduction as good,
75 per cent reduction as very good and 100 per cent as excellent.
In 45 per cent or 18 of his cases he achieved very good results,
in another 18 cases he achieved good results and in only 4 cases
were the results classified as slight.

Barbara Cartland, who is surely one of the most attractive women
of her age in the world, has written many words in praise of *Melbrosia PLD* and of pollen. She is not only glamorous, but also
exceptionally hard working. In her 76th year she wrote 24 books,
all of them best sellers! And now, fit and vibrant in her 80s, she
still writes at least 12 books every year. She has found that *Melbrosia* works for her and for countless men and women who need
to retain vigour, beauty and vitality.

Chapter 7

VIRILITY AND REJUVENATION

'Everyman desires to live long: but no man would be old.' —
Swift 1714

It is fashionable to sneer at or make light of any form of rejuvenation. Yet health should be the normal state of man, and the
fact of the matter is that a man can and does retain his virility
and a woman her sexuality when the undernourished and tired
body is restored to normality.

Convenience foods made for the convenience of the manufac-
turer rather than the consumer, lack of sensible and wise cook-
ing of good basic raw materials, the excessive dependence upon
tranquillizers, sedatives and strong stimulants — these factors,
together with too much smoking, too little exercise and even too
little excitement with the joy of life itself — all contribute to the
unnecessarily early degeneration of our bodies.

Yet how difficult it is to escape from our inadequate and sub-
standard way of living. The housewife finds that she has to snatch
a hurried lunch in order to have enough time to cope with the
daily tasks. Too much tea laden with sugar is drunk. Factory or
office, businessmen or labourers all suffer pressures forcing them
to live on wrong foods in unhealthy atmospheres — surely good
health need not be such a struggle!

As we get older it is often the case that many of the nutrients
necessary for good health become difficult to assimilate. Because
of the remarkable phenomenon of persorption, pollen does seem
to be particularly well assimilated so that all the many vitamins,
amino acids, minerals and micro-nutrients present are able to enter

the blood-stream straight from the stomach itself. Certainly it is with older people that some of the most remarkable trials with pollen have been achieved. But even younger men and women with cohabitation difficulties have been remarkably improved, so transforming the very lives of people who have begun to feel truly inadequate.

POLLEN FOR POTENCY

In 1977 Professor Osmanagic published a scientific paper summarizing the results of his trials with *Melbrosia Executive*, a particularly strong blend of pollen and royal jelly, on 40 men.

He noted that sexual impotence in men is far more frequent than is generally thought, as many men are reluctant to consult a doctor about their problems. Contact was established with the patients studied in his report through the person most concerned about a man's impotence — his wife! These women consulted the Gynaecological Clinic at The University of Sarajevo about the infertility of their marriages. It was discovered that, in many cases, it was not the woman to blame, as is so often assumed, but the man.

Impotence is usually understood as the inability to carry out sexual intercourse, so he was surprised to find that a large number of his patients were actually suffering from poor sperm production. Although a man's potency is most often judged by his ability to carry out the act, fertilization is the most necessary part of the concept of potency.

A reduction or even a complete lack of potency can be caused by glandular, nervous or psychological disturbances. These are very often related to one another because there are close connections between sexual functions, hormonal activities, and the central nervous system. Because of this, hormonal and psychological problems often occur together.

Psychologically the man can suffer anxiety and fear as to whether the intercourse will be successful. He may also find that he just does not have enough interest in his partner.

Sterility in man can on the other hand have physical origins and these must also be taken into account. So Professor Osmanagic studied his patients with regard to not only their ability to cohabit with their wives but also their actual powers of fertilization.

The men he studied were between 20 and 52 years of age and, with a few exceptions, were mostly skilled or semi-skilled. They had all had sterile marriages for two or more years. After being questioned about their economic situation, way of life, sexual habits and the conditions of their marriage, they were evaluated systematically through questioning and through laboratory clinical examinations. The velocity, motility and form of the sperms were examined to see if the treatment had produced any positive changes.

Professor Osmanagic concluded that 75 per cent of his patients were suffering from sperm deficiency. They took two capsules a day of *Melbrosia Executive* and each had either 80 or 160 capsules in all. During the course of the two or three months treatment the patients were interviewed at least three times and the sperm count repeated. Undesirable side-effects were not observed in any of the patients.

After just one month more than half (57.5 per cent) showed an improvement in their general and sexual condition with a significant effect on their self-confidence. A quarter found that the quality of their cohabitation had improved and the majority showed improved sperm production. Two patients were delighted to announce that their wives were now pregnant — astounding proof of the effectiveness of this treatment as these fertilizations were made by so-called 'infertile' men.

In summary, 22.5 per cent of the patients achieved a very good result, 37.5 per cent a good result and 27.5 per cent a poor result (12.5 per cent did not return for re-examination).

Professor Osmanagic concluded that the treatment with *Melbrosia Executive* led to an improvement in the general state of health, an increase in sexual activity and improved sperm production. He went on to say that this represents proof of the positive effect of the product in cases of reduced sexual and procreative potency.

137 YEARS OLD — STILL WORKING

You will have read of those areas of the world where people grow to a great age. In the village of Kutoli in the Ochamchir district of the Abkhazian Autonomous Republic a splendid old lady of 137, Khfaf Lazuria, was still working until she died at the age of 139 in 1975, when she was thought to be the oldest woman in the world.

In September 1978, the *British Medical Journal* published a study into the lives, physical conditions and habits of a large group of Dutch people who were all over 90 years old. The one common factor seemed to be that only 2 per cent smoked. In Georgia, the old people do not usually smoke. They also take a lot of unstrained honey rich in pollen. In order to enjoy a youthful old age it may be necessary to work hard during the early part of your life, to eat fresh good natural foods without too much fat and to live in an unpolluted area taking plenty of unstrained honey all your life. For most of us it is too late to do this or just plain impossible. But the good news is that pollen really does seem to help, as does royal jelly, a good proportion of older people.

FRENCH GOVERNMENT CONSULTANT APPROVES POLLEN PRODUCT

Dr Jacques DuBrisay is a Paris consultant to the French Ministry of Social Affairs. He carried out an extensive trial on a Cernelle pollen product called *Amplamil*. This is a capsule containing 6 mg of fat-soluble and 120 mg of water-soluble pollen extract. Before undertaking this test he carefully studied previous French reports which had verified that pollen was safe to take.

He took 48 men patients and divided them into two random groups, A and B. Then he divided the capsules and identical looking placebo capsules into two further groups also called A and B. Neither the patients nor the physician knew which type of capsule was being given to either group. All these men were chronic cases who had been residential patients in hospital for several months before the trial began. Dr DuBrisay used the so-called double-blind technique so that no one knew who was receiving which treatment in order that the psychological factors often present in conditions of the elderly were ruled out.

The patients were chosen because they had considerable loss of appetite and had no real desire to eat. They also suffered from both mental and physical exhaustion. The average age of group A was 70 and of group B 72. The men received four capsules a day for four weeks.

Blood pressure was checked twice weekly and no changes were observed — a good result as one has to be very careful about increasing blood pressure in the old. There were no untoward side-effects of any sort and even patients who were prone to asthmatic attacks showed no intolerance. The blood, liver and kidney functions were all carefully observed without any disorder resulting.

When assessing the results the good doctor strongly emphasized that the general weakness and loss of appetite was severe in every case. All were elderly and living alone, many had lost the will to live. Results were rated 'very good', 'good', 'fair', 'poor', or 'nil'.

The results in group A, who had the genuine capsules, were:
very good: 13 = 54.17 per cent
good: 10 = 41.66 per cent
fair: 1 = 4.17 per cent.

These results were clearly positive since 23 patients responded well to treatment. Indeed, the poor result obtained in the single 'fair' case was open to doubt because of another condition which developed during the treatment.

Group B received the imitation capsules. Their results were:
fair: 3 = 12.5 per cent
poor: 11 = 45.84 per cent
nil: 10 = 41.66 per cent.

So the positive results were *all* in the group receiving pollen.

The conditions which the treatment with pollen helped to cure included many of those afflictions which are distressing to the old and even more distressing to those who must look after them, including general weariness, apathy, wishing for death, listlessness, and in some cases no wish to leave the bed or to dress, loss of interest in reading and rejection of all contact with the environment.

FATIGUE RELIEVED

The patients were also given tests which were evaluated by statisticians in order to see whether the treatment had any effect on fatigue, appetite, weight gain, blood cholesterol, total energy, concentration and speed, as well as many of the chemically checkable functions of the body.

Results were astonishing; taking a substantial improvement as the indication of a good result, fatigue resistance was greatly improved in 83.3 per cent of cases in group A and in no cases in group B. Appetite was greatly improved in 75 per cent in group A and in no cases in group B.

Both groups had approximately the same average weight at the beginning of the four-week treatment period but by the end, although group B had shown no improvement at all, group A had increased in weight by almost 7 lb (3.271 kg) — exactly the result that would do the most good for these old people. The tests for energy and strength, for concentration, and for speed of performance all showed very significant improvements. That group of old people were able to look life in the face and live again!

Dr DuBrisay concluded that the pollen product was therapeutically useful, has no harmful effects, and that it qualifies for a visa under article L.601 of the Public Health Code.

Wassen, the makers of *Pollen-B*, have been carrying out long-term clinical trials with their tablets at an English hospital, in order to give added support to the many letters they have received from users reporting a reduction in fatigue in the older person. They have no doubt, from all the information available, that the trials will provide yet more scientific evidence to support the experience of countless satisfied users.

Ortis of Belgium have also amassed much more evidence from all over Europe from users of their pollen preparations, and our study of these confirms the finding that for the great majority of men and women who have lost the pleasure, excitement and joy of life, pollen therapy represents an effective, safe and long-term remedy which is able to truly rejuvenate the human organism.

Chapter 8

CHILDREN

'Children bring with them innumerable cares.' — Erasmus 1522

Child health must begin at the beginning. There is now ample evidence to show that breast feeding contributes greatly to sound health and a good constitution. It is now generally realized that solids, especially cereals, should not be given before the twelfth week. This is because there is a small but definite risk of an adverse reaction, a risk usually passed by the third month. Some women simply cannot breast feed or they may have children who were not breast fed. In such cases second to best just has to be good enough.

The next important aspect is diet. We know what should be done, but do we do it? The average person eats far too much fat, salt, sugar and refined foods, and not enough roughage, whole grains, lightly cooked or raw fruit and vegetables. Give your child a good start by ensuring a sensible and balanced diet, avoiding anything more than the occasional sweet or sugary soft drink, making doubly certain that fond relatives and friends do not use sweets as a reward. Eat sensibly yourself — example is better than mere words and avoid smoking (especially during pregnancy and lactation). Alcohol is now known to have a detrimental effect on the developing foetus and should only be taken in very modest amounts.

Add fresh air, exercise, sunshine, a stable loving home life and plenty of fun and companionship. For most children such simple steps as these are sufficient to reduce to the minimum the likelihood of childhood illness. In spite of a good deal of backsliding of all concerned and without taking it all too seriously, such a philosophy can help to keep children relatively free from illness and exhaustingly full of energy.

Inevitably things do go wrong. Epidemics occur at school. The sun doesn't shine all summer, or hardly seems to, so that resistance is reduced. Visits to exhibitions or concerts, rides on trains and buses, all seem sometimes to be part of a gigantic plot to expose the family to germs which seem to have left their producers in a catastrophic state.

Of course, there will be times when everything fails and rest in bed is the only answer. But the secret of a good deal of success is to take up battle stations as soon as there is a risk of serious infection. And here the bee comes to the rescue and is part of our defences. A two or three months' course of pollen in the autumn, especially if the summer has been bad, is a wise and effective precaution. The evidence that pollen also aids concentration could be an added bonus at school!

But when danger really threatens and the children are exposed to many germs, then, at the first sign of distress — however slight — give vitamin C (natural if possible) at least 300 to 500 mg a day together with one or two capsules or lozenges a day of propolis, the bee resin described fully later, and if there is anything more than the slightest symptoms step up the vitamin C for children over the age of 10 to a gram three or four times a day and when over the age of 15 to a gram every three hours for at least two days (not necessary at night).

At the same time increase the propolis to three or four capsules a day. If you can find propolis tincture then take five drops in a glass of water, gargle with it and swallow the mixture at the first signs of a sore throat. Propolis and vitamin C are, like pollen, very useful in all infectious illnesses and are not contra-indicated by any other treatment that is being given by your practitioner (although it is sensible to let him or her know what you are doing). Even when it does not completely clear up the illness, this treatment has been shown to help keep the symptoms reasonably mild in the majority of cases.

HAY FEVER

Children tend to suffer from hay fever far more frequently than adults and it is certainly worthwhile reading the chapter on hay fever and giving pollen a good trial, preferably over two years. Another excellent hay fever treatment which can be used as well as pollen and is often dramatically swift in the relief of symptoms is *Combination H*, a biochemic tissue salt mixture which has been homoeopathically prepared and is quite safe even for the youngest child.

WHEAT GERM AND POLLEN SACHETS

Some people, especially children and the old, find tablets and capsules difficult to take. After two years of research there are now delicious sachets of wheat germ with pollen made by the *Pollen-B (Bee Pollen from England)* company. These are produced by a special cold process which preserves the enzymes whilst protecting the granules.

Chapter 9

MORE USES FOR POLLEN

'Life is not just living, but living in health.' — Martial A.D.90

Because pollen balances the body so effectively, it is not surprising that the many micro-nutrients present exert a beneficial effect on many illnesses and psychological states. We are only beginning to scratch the surface in our search for nature's remedies, but without doubt man's understanding of honey, propolis, royal jelly and pollen will continue to increase and grow in importance.

DIABETES

Dr Rudolf Frey, who is the head physician of the Korneuburg hospital in Austria, reported on the effect of a pollen product rich in royal jelly made by Melbrosin to see whether it would alleviate the problems often faced by diabetics. It was not the purpose or even a possibility of the trial that it could cure the actual diabetes. Pollen preparations are not in any way a substitute for insulin or the other substances which help diabetic people. Also, the use of the preparation did not have any effect on the treatment for the condition so that it was a true supplement without any actual effect on the diabetes itself but, as it turned out, with remarkable benefits in helping the control of many side-effects.

Apart from an increased liability to infection, the complications of diabetes principally involve conditions of the vascular system. Dr Frey found that the product was especially effective in the case of diabetics who were not particularly well-adjusted to their treatment and showed signs of mental and physical exhaustion.

In addition, difficulties with walking, decline of mental and physical powers, menstrual problems, sleeplessness, rheumatic conditions, forgetfulness and lack of concentration, circulatory disorders and chronic constipation were all included in the complaints that responded most favourably to the treatment.

Pollen and royal jelly preparations were given every morning half an hour before breakfast on an empty stomach over a period of 21 days. It seems that all pollen preparations are most effective when taken this way, on a completely empty stomach. Sometimes it was found necessary to begin a second course some eight to ten days after the conclusion of the first one.

Dr Frey gave some interesting case histories of some of his patients. For example one patient, who was 48 years old, had suffered from diabetes since he was 18 and had taken daily injections of sixty units of insulin for 30 years. He had perfectly adjusted to his insulin and his diet and was able to work as a lorry driver. However, he had suffered for eight months from intermittent claudication, which meant that he could not walk more than 50 yards without experiencing violent cramp in the calves of his legs forcing him to stop. Preparations were given to improve the supply of blood to the legs and to help the nervous system, but his condition was only slightly improved by these normal therapeutic measures. Nevertheless, after two courses of a treatment with the Melbrosin product the patient felt much better, his general feeling of depression gave way to a feeling of pleasure, the pain in the calves lessened and at last the patient was able to walk again without the occurrence of cramps.

Another patient, a 35-year-old housewife and mother of two children, had suffered from diabetes for only two years, but had adjusted to the condition very well and was taking twenty units of insulin daily. But two children and the care of the house were a great strain, especially to a diabetic, and she was mentally and physically exhausted, complained of forgetfulness and sleeplessness and in the last months was no longer able to carry out her household duties. She was given sedatives and then tonics but there was no noticeable improvement. After two courses of pollen and royal jelly treatment she was able to sleep normally once more, her tiredness disappeared very rapidly and she was once again able to perform her usual duties as a happy housewife and fond mother.

Diabetes sometimes begins in old age. This was the case of a 71-year-old gentleman who had hardening of the arteries and had complained of great thirst for more than a year. An examination showed that he was suffering from mild diabetes which was controllable by attention to the diet. But as time went past he began to suffer from forgetfulness which rapidly increased in degree, and he also experienced a pronounced failing of his powers of concentration. Since he had always been a person used to brain-work this sudden diminution of his mental powers brought him to the verge of a nervous breakdown, all the more because the medicines prescribed by his doctor, and on which he had based his hopes, did not help him in the least. A course of injections was also tried and this had no result. Indeed, it was not until the patient had taken two courses of pollen and royal jelly treatment that he began to regain his strength and to lose his strong tendency towards forgetfulness. The result was that he could once again concentrate and continue to enjoy life as he had done before.

A similar case was a 35-year-old sales manager in a fashion store who found himself unable to work because of his loss of concentration and forgetfulness resulting from his diabetic condition. Here again a six-week treatment with pollen and royal jelly restored him to his usual active self.

Dr Frey concluded from his experience of these and many other cases that a good preperation of pollen and royal jelly was a completely harmless natural remedy without any allergic after-effects. He believed that the high concentration of royal jelly combined with pollen with their content of trace elements and glutamic acid (an important substance with regard to the metabolism of the nucleus) combined together to achieve very good results in connection with the various disorders which often follow diabetes. He fully justified their use and recommended administration as a general treatment.

STRESS, ANXIETY AND DEPRESSION

Words such as stress, anxiety and depression mean different things to different people. To the psychiatrist they represent conditions that are often serious, requiring much medical patience and skill to overcome. We have seen that, under medical supervision, certain pollen products have indeed been shown to be effective in helping patients with quite distressing mental conditions.

How pollen does this is not at all clear. Some researchers believe that pollen and royal jelly exert a mutually beneficial effect upon each other, thus giving results better than either do individually; but the work of Cernelle in Sweden has produced excellent results without royal jelly.

There may be quite wide variations in the individual response to the treatment with pollen and, of course, pollens differ quite considerably in their individual content of substances, so it is quite possible that in certain cases that which is lacking in a particular pollen can be made up for in the royal jelly. We shall have to wait and see the answer to these and many more questions regarding pollen but one thing is quite clear. Pollen and royal jelly are both safe to take and for a lot of people they help to strengthen the body, guard against infection and lift the shadows of anxiety and depression.

We are all over-stressed at some time or another; we all have moments of anxiety; indeed, of desperation; and these often lead us to times of depression when those closest to us have to make allowances for our behaviour.

It is not very surprising that this inability to cope with the normal problems of life could well be due to dietary deficiencies, perhaps in those trace elements which are required in incredibly small quantities by our bodies. The latest research into trace elements has shown that chromium, tin, vanadium, fluorine, silicon and nickel are all necessary for higher animals, and we are certainly among those! Often the dietary concentrations required are less than one part in a million.

Recently there has been a considerable amount of research into the value of zinc and selenium, which, although highly toxic in great amounts, nevertheless have, in minute doses, a role to play in maintaining our bodies in good order. It may be that many of those conditions including nervous disorders where pollen seems so effective are due to the persorption phenomenon allowing the micro-nutrients in pollen to be absorbed when they are failing to be taken in from normal foods.

The conclusion is clear and straightforward. When life, people and events begin to get on top of you, try a two-month course of pollen therapy and see if it works as well for you as it has for many of the cases that are described in this book. You may not be able to solve life's problems, but at least you will be able to deal with them.

Chapter 10

POLLEN POWER FOR ATHLETES

'You're on the right track.' — Plautus 200 B.C.

Pollen has an amazing and well proved effect upon athletic performance. Pollen power is not just a headline — it is a fact. Men and women undergoing the rigours of athletic training notice the slightest differences in their fitness; differences which we ordinary mortals could not possibly imagine. For a great race the perfectly prepared athlete is as finely tuned as a Stradivarius violin. Even ordinary school and club athletes record substantial benefits after taking pollen: it helps them all, the perfectly fit and the weekend sportsman.

Many distinguished coaches and international athletes have spoken of the positive results that they had experienced following regular supplementation with pollen.

Pollen may be regarded as being part of the ideal athlete's diet, i.e. that diet pattern which produces the maximum performance when it is required and has no long-term harmful side-effects. It is tragic that the increased use of harmful drugs such as anabolic steroids and pep pills — drugs that can destroy the athlete's health and in the case of steroids sometimes cause cancer and loss of potency in men — occurs in the name of success, when the athlete should be taking a diet composed of entirely natural and beneficial products and supplements which also produce magnificent results but have none of the harmful dangers.

Everything that goes into your mouth, or even in certain cases through the skin, is part of the diet that has nutritional consequences. Your body is being continually renewed and the average half-life (which is the time taken for half to be replaced) of protein, for example, in the body is 80 days. But the time differs with different tissues. For blood serum, heart, liver and kidneys it is 10 days, while for bone, skin and muscle it is 158 days. The other constituents of your body are, for the most part, also replaced continually by what you consume.

For this reason it is vitally important that an athlete's diet is always soundly based. It is simply not good enough to eat correctly for part of the year only — it is the *quantity* that needs to be altered at times of lesser or greater activity, not the quality. However, several research workers have demonstrated that an increase in the consumption of fructose (fruit sugar), before an event helps to build up reserves of energy when this is done in controlled form.

POLLEN TESTS FOR SPORTSMEN

Cernelle organized major symposia on the effect of pollen for athletes in 1972 in Sweden and in 1973 in London. The Swedish meeting was notable for a report on *Pollitabs* used by nine doctors attached to nine important Italian football teams. The teams were divided between professional, semi-professional, and amateur footballers, and they set out to test whether *Pollitabs* given for 30 days produced any real immediate benefit and whether they had lasting good effects in both the short and medium term.

The doctors recorded changes in the players' physical condition, condition of breathing, and physical resistance. This was also related to the number of days of training and play. Conclusions were that in almost all the cases the general state of health was improved, together with substantial improvements in the players' breathing and their physical resistance to sporting fatigue. One exception was the team called Mantova where at the start of the experiment the state of fitness of the players was so perfect that no improvement was measurable!

The effect of the pollen consumption was progressive. The greatest percentage change takes place between the second and third 10-day periods. They also confirmed that the *Pollitabs* did not cause any undesirable side-effects whatsoever. Dr Coronelli considered the validity of the test to be beyond question.

Other researchers related the extraordinary effects of pollen to the micro-nutrients present. This view was much supported by new information at the Trace Element Conference held in Aberdeen between 27 and 29 June 1978. Dr Neil T. Davies, of the Rowett Research Institute, viewed the current situation on chromium, tin, vanadium, fluorine, silicon and nickel which are essential for animals. He said that with the exception of silicon, these elements are required at dietary concentrations of one part per million or less. Tin, for example, has a beneficial effect on the growth rate.

The extraordinary richness of pollen in these micro-elements cannot be stressed too much. We just cannot be sure that a normal diet produces enough in an available form so the persorption properties of pollen allow the trace elements to be incorporated into the body's structure without excessive loss.

POLLEN AT THE OLYMPICS
The bees helped back Britain in the Montreal Olympics. Geoff Capes, the shot putter; Andrea Lynch and Donna Murray, the sprinters; and Bill Hartley, the hurdler, are just four of the star athletes who found that pollen which bees collected from flowers helped to maintain peak fitness. The *Glasgow Herald* reported that Tom McNab, the National Athletics Coach, was among those convinced that daily pollen tablets build strength and energy as well as warding off colds and other infections which can interrupt an athlete's training or affect performance.

McNab was especially impressed, says the *Herald*, by the experience of the Finns, who had managed to put only one runner among the top 100 in the last but one Olympics but with the help of *Pollitabs* had boosted that score to a remarkable 39 at Munich four years later. The British athletes were all reported to be using *Pollen-B. Pollitabs* were also used in very many cases.

When the Finns were reporting the results of their experiments with pollen, they said they believed that the lack of trace elements in today's average diet, which made pollen such a necessity, was due to intensive farming, big crops, strong fertilizers, use of cattle manure, altered soil factors, absence of equilibrium between macro- and micro-nutrients, processed products used as cattle feed, and finally the poor preparation and conservation of food-stuffs.

It was clear that the Finns believed pollen was a key factor in protecting man from the modern environment in which he is forced to live. To conquer the diseases of western civilization it now looks as if we do not just need plenty of wholemeal bread but would do well to combine that with regular courses of pollen.

EARLY TRIALS
One of the earliest trials was done way back in 1961 in Florida by Dr Noyes who reported that during the previous two years he had used *Pollitabs* in his practice for many diverse complaints and syndromes. Certain results, he said, occurred predominantly regardless of the purpose for which the tablet was prescribed. Foremost among these have been increased appetite, weight gain, increased vigour and sense of well-being, and decreased susceptibility to infection. Therefore it was thought that a football team would make a good preliminary controlled study to determine these factors in an objective manner, i.e. weight gain and resistance to infection.

He therefore selected a local high school football team, consisting of 30 active players, and divided them into two groups, those receiving *Pollitabs* and those receiving a standard multi-vitamin preparation. The study covered a period of 15 weeks in which for the first three neither product was used. It was during this initial three-week period that each player lost excessive weight, in most cases representing excess fat.

At the end of the third week 15 players were started on two *Pollitabs* a day and the control group on the multi-vitamins daily. All medication was administered daily and individually by the coach. The group taking *Pollitabs* regained their pre-season weight after taking the tablets for 7½ weeks, and 4½ weeks later at the end of the season the Pollitabs group actually showed a 5½ lb (2½ kilo) average increase in weight over their pre-season level.

The group taking the multi-vitamins remained generally constant from the third to fifteenth week showing no further loss or gain. The opinion was expressed by impartial former professional players that it is almost unheard of for a football player to weigh more at the end of a season than he did before practice started.

Infections were also dramatically reduced. During the whole season the *Pollitabs* group of 15 boys lost between them five playing days because of flu and one playing day because of colds. The boys who took the multi-vitamins lost 16 playing days because of colds and 18 because of flu.

'ALI'S MAGIC POTION'

Britain's four million copy circulation newspaper, *The Sunday Mirror*, blazed the 'Ali's Magic Potion' banner headline across the front page as the main news item on 24 September 1978. 'Now it can be told,' they said. 'Mohammed Ali swallowed a secret potion before he won the world heavyweight championship for a record third time.

'Ali, 36, astounded the world by his vitality and staying power and outclassed 25-year-old Leon Spinks in New Orleans nine days ago.

'The potion — a kind of vitamin cocktail — was invented by a Dr Alvenia Fulton, a Chicago nutrition expert who although she is 70 is still trim enough to wear a bikini on the beach.' Philip Finn, the *Mirror's* New York reporter, went on to give details of her special formula which included vitamin E, magnesium, bee pollen tablets, folic acid, lecithin, vitamin B6 together with honey, all crushed and mixed with orange juice which also contains vitamin C.

Ali had spoken about the potion after his fight in New Orleans and again when he returned home to Chicago. He said: 'It was a great mixture and I danced and danced and tired Spinks out.' Ali took the potion on the advice of his friend, comedian Dick Gregory, who has known Dr Fulton for years. Dr Fulton, who runs a health food centre in Chicago, said: 'Dick contacted me on the afternoon of the fight to check what was best to give Ali. I recommended the mixture. Vitamins plus particularly the magnesium put more oxygen into the bloodstream to give extra wind and stamina. Anyone who saw Mohammed fight must have noticed how he got stronger and stronger. He could have gone on dancing and fighting all night. He defied all the so-called experts who said he was too old at 36. I am convinced that if Ali continues to follow my advice he will go on fighting — and winning — for another five years.'

This fantastic performance came after Mohammed Ali had lost to Spinks in Las Vegas the previous February. Those who saw him were amazed at his condition and fitness for this return fight. What is more, he broke no rules by taking the vitamin and pollen cocktail. As Dr Adrian Whiteson, who is the Chief Medical Adviser to the British Boxing Board of Control, said: 'Vitamins are not drugs. They are not stimulants — and there would be nothing to stop any boxer taking them before a fight. But they would not be allowed in the boxer's corner.'

So the secret of Ali's amazing come-back had bee pollen tablets as a key ingredient.

SWEDISH COURTS SUPPORT POLLEN FOR SPORTSMEN

Advertising laws covering any product which makes a claim for health or fitness vary from country to country and even from place to place, and are a jungle. It is often very difficult to tell the consumers the truth about a natural food supplement which is in any way out of the normal run of things. Pollen for sportsmen certainly is in that category.

A Swedish court had to settle a case when an advertisement in one of the largest Swedish daily papers, *Dagbladet,* appeared almost by mistake when a secretary accidentally confirmed a cancelled order. The advertisement said: 'Do as the Finns, increase your performance capacity by taking Cernelle pollen tablets.' The consumer information bureaucrats called it 'inappropriate marketing' and demanded prohibition under penalty of a fine for Cernelle because they used this text. So Cernelle took the case to court.

Many expert witnesses spoke in defence of the Cernelle process which had been developed more than a quarter of a century before in which, as Professor Olov Lindahl said: 'The essence is manufactured from the very core substance of the pollen grains and con-

tains in small quantities all known vitamins, all trace minerals, some albumen, and all known amino acids.'

These substances may indeed have a good effect on the human body, but probably it is other unidentified parts of the pollen core that have the effect observed. Professor Lindahl's opinion was that the pollen preparations are healing and have a medical effect; however, in this case, it was not a question of the registration of the pollen tablets as pharmaceutical preparations, but of pollen as a food supplement.

The officials were also upset with the picture of three runners that appeared with the advertisement because it featured the Finn Lasse Viren's famous run at the Munich Olympics in which he stumbled and fell but picked himself up again to win the 10,000 metre gold medal.

Viren, like 70 per cent of the Finn runners, used pollen when training. Pollen has the proven ability of really increasing the performance capacity, the perseverance and the power. A pollen runner can train up to 50 kilometres a day instead of the normal 30 kilometres and he does not need the 5,000 daily calories that a top sportsman usually consumes. These are all important factors when you are running against the best in the world.

Pollen is not a drug like the anabolic steroids used with personal danger by so many athletes; it is not against any rules or regulations; and indeed it is not a miraculous medicine, it is just a valuable and a natural product. That is why there is great interest among sports people in the increased use of pollen supplements.

In support of their case against Cernelle the authorities said that they had rejected registration of all natural medicines because the scientific material handed over was not sufficient to prove the effect of the product. It was pointed out that they were not claiming pollen to be a medicine but the authorities said the same arguments stood — the claims were misleading and inappropriate.

Cernelle showed them the many important clinical trials that had taken place on pollen which you will find elsewhere in this book. It was calculated that the results obtained by Professor DuBrisay in improving the condition of old people were statistically phenomenal.

In social or psychological science one star significance is enough as a proof of the effect, that is to say the chance that an accidentally good result has occurred is five in a hundred. In medicine they are satisfied with two star proof where the chance is one in a thousand. A medicine can often be registered on this basis.

In the French examination of 48 patients the chance that they could have got better independently of the pollen preparation was only one chance in one million million. In medical terms that means that the significance has eleven stars and is an extraordinary proof of the pollen preparations.

Professor Lindahl in his summary concluded that pollen preparations can be used to treat diseases, improve sports performances, increase working capacity and diminish tiredness in people. His opinion was supported by the statisticians Lars Lindwall and Arne Sandström.

The authorities did not give up. They found a doctor who had the opposite opinion! An argument ensued between Lindahl and Dr Hellström and the fight went on. The medical authorities in Sweden even tried to cast doubt on the very high qualifications and ability of Professor DuBrisay. DuBrisay was a professor in experimental medicine with an examination qualification much higher than most of those examinations which are the basis for being entitled to investigate pharmaceutical preparations in Sweden.

Lindahl once again drew attention to a place in the French report where it showed that one of the patients who had had a very slow-healing fracture healed with remarkable speed as soon as pollen therapy was tried. In fact, the cases of the 265 French patients who had been given pollen therapy had not been critically examined at all by the Swedish Welfare Board who had simply ignored the important French clinical trial.

The courts summary filled forty sheets of closely argued conclusions with the result that Cernelle was given permission to advertise as they had done before and were fully supported by the court. The important and far-reaching result of this case is that in January 1978 far greater freedom was given for the produc-

tion, sale and advertising of natural medicines in Sweden than had been the case there for very many years. It seems that pollen does not just help cure people — it changes the minds of governments!

Chapter 11

AN INTRODUCTION TO PROPOLIS

'That which is not good for the swarm, neither is it good for the bee.' — Marcus Aurelius A.D. 174

Although much of this book is about pollen, we share with Paul Urban of Melbrosin and the Horn family of Ortis the belief that propolis, the sweet-smelling resin used by the bees as a sealing compound in their hives, will soon be thought of as a major medical breakthrough, perhaps even as important as the discovery of penicillin. The World Health Organization is also investigating propolis because it is believed to be a safe, natural antibiotic.

Medical opinion in those centres of research where propolis has been investigated during the past few years has altered from one of complete cynicism to the enthusiastic use of propolis for many different illnesses. In future, many may benefit from their exciting discoveries.

Take, for example, Mitja Vosnjak. He is no ordinary man. His meteoric rise in the Yugoslav Diplomatic Corps led him from being Deputy Minister of Foreign Affairs to the post of Ambassador to East Germany and then on to become Ambassador of Austria in the romantic capital, Vienna.

He found that his demanding life as a diplomat, poet, and novelist was taking a heavy toll on his health. He felt that boundless reserves of vitality that had stood him in such good stead in times of stress and crisis were ebbing away in the prime of his life, and what was more his eyesight was failing.

Then he met Paul Urban, who told him of the discoveries that had been made for improving health with the products of the bees, and in spite of his doubt at such an idea he started on a course of *Melbrosia for Men*, a mixture of pollen and royal jelly.

He found that his failure in health and eyesight were both restored because of the micro-nutrients present in pollen and he became so excited that he gave up his distinguished career and began a new life devoted to finding out more about the bees.

Since 1974, as the Director of the Centre for Biotic Research, he has interested many distinguished scientists from many lands in the subject of api-therapy (the medical application of bee products). Discovery led to discovery. Propolis, he found, was perhaps the first non-toxic anti-infective agent. Today this one-time ambassador and honorary general of the army quietly continues what has become his life's quest.

A SHORT HISTORY OF ITS USE

Propolis is a resinous mixture used by bees to protect the hive against intruders. These unwanted invaders may be large, such as a mouse or lizard, or small, such as germs. Propolis is effective against them all, and numerous medical and scientific research studies have confirmed the amazing values of this material.

The human race has been aware of the benefits of propolis for thousands of years. The ancient Egyptians, and later the Greeks and the Romans, all used propolis for healing. There is even a legend that the god Jupiter changed the beautiful Melissa into a bee so she could become a provider of the healing material.

Hippocrates (460-377 B.C.), known to us as the 'father of medicine', recorded his use of propolis as an ointment to treat wounds, sores and ulcers. Around four hundred years later, the Roman scholar Pliny extolled the values of the resin. He referred to propolis in a number of his writings, explaining how it 'extracts stings and all substances embedded in the flesh, reduces swelling, softens hardened areas, soothes pain of the sinews and heals sores when it appears hopeless for them to mend'.

Between the eleventh and fifteenth centuries the use of propolis was recorded in medical books in Georgia. For example, it was described as a device against infections of the mouth cavity, swelling and against dental decay. It was recommended to help remove corns and to treat colds and rheumatic pains. There was also a custom of placing a small amount on the navel of newborn babies.

Moving on through history we reach the seventeenth century, when the famous herbalist, Nicholas Culpeper, stated 'the ointment called propolis is singularly good for all heat and inflammations in any part of the body, and tempers the heat of wounds'. This leads us straight to the beginning of the twentieth century and the Boer War. During the three years of the battle (1899-1902), the modern treatments of the day were in desperately short supply. Therapy reverted to the traditional, with dried moss as absorptive dressings and propolis, made into an ointment with petroleum jelly, as an effective wound healer.

PROPOLIS IN THE BEEHIVE

The word propolis is composed of the Greek *pro* meaning before or in front of and *polis* meaning city. Propolis is the material used by the bees to maintain their hive as a fortified city. The bees use propolis as a cement, to make the entrance to the hive smaller in order to prevent the entry of predators. The astonishing fact is that if an enemy does manage to sneak in, the bees will also use propolis to embalm the body after stinging it to death. This behaviour was noted by the Danish scientist K. Lund Aagaard in the 1950s in his home village of Helsinge. One day Aagaard found the mummified body of a perfectly preserved mouse on the floor of one of his hives. He deduced that the mouse must have been there for a number of months and yet it showed none of the expected signs of decay.

Bees are astonishingly clean insects. They keep the hive free of germs and, unlike other animals, are resistant to bacterial and viral infections. Professor Remy Chauvin of Paris carried out a study looking at the external infestations of various animals and noted that bees were the only ones that were entirely free of bacterial colonies. He found this surprising and went on to discover that propolis is the anti-bacterial agent. The bees use propolis as an all-purpose disinfectant, as well as being a useful cement. Each cell in the comb is treated with propolis prior to the queen laying her eggs, and the walls of the hive are coated with the substance (this acts as an insulator as well as a disinfectant). This means that the hive is more sterile than the average hospital, quite an achievement for an insect that has been around for 40 million years, and one that lives packed in with 50,000 neighbours.

HOW BEES COLLECT PROPOLIS

Propolis is made up of the resinous exudate from the buds and bark of trees. The bees only collect this resin at certain times of the year, and prefer the sunniest days as this makes the material softer and easier to break off. Observers in Germany noted that the favoured months for collection are August, September and October, although activity does commence in June. The favoured time of day is between 10 a.m. and 3.30 p.m., again making the best use of the warmth of the sun.

When the bee finds a good piece of material suitable for propolis she breaks it off with her jaws and chews it gently to soften it further. She then transfers it to the pollen baskets on her back legs, ready for the flight home. Once back inside the hive she settles quietly near the outer walls and waits for other bees to come and remove what they need for their work. Each bee takes a small amount and uses it for cementing gaps, repair or for preparation or disinfecting, as required. The process of emptying the pollen baskets of propolis may take several hours, with one hour as the minimum.

The ingredients of propolis will vary according to the type of tree in the vicinity of the hive and the climate. The bees search out trees such as poplar. birch, chestnut and oak and find the blobs of sticky resin that the trees manufacture to keep off pests. These very resins have a history of medicinal use for human disorders. In Green's *Universal Herbal* of 1824, the buds of the poplar tree are described as yielding 'a resinous substance' used in healing 'internal ulcers and cuts'.

The man whose interest in propolis was aroused by the embalmed mouse, K. Lund Aagaard, went off to devote 20 years to studying the substance and its effects. He stressed the importance of the bees' collecting propolis from areas rich in tree life and yet free of man's insecticides. After all, the resin is the trees' own protector and the addition of other chemicals will only pollute this natural substance. K. Lund Aagaard's studies were so lengthy and detailed that he became known as 'Mr Propolis'.

HARVESTING PROPOLIS

Mr Propolis likened the harvesting of the material to the collection of grapes for wine. There is a prime season for the production of the best grade, and the correct procedures of extraction must be followed in order to maintain the characteristics of the product.

When the propolis is first removed from the hive it is soft, sticky and aromatic and tastes burningly bitter. It tends to have an aroma of birch or poplar buds or of honey or vanilla. Its colour may be brown, dark green, grey or even tending towards black. In order to provide a consistent product the propolis from various sources is generally blended. With this blending treatment you can be sure of getting good quality all the time.

The treatment and storage of propolis after harvesting are important. Being aromatic and susceptible to heat, the propolis must be treated gently. It is carefully cleaned after collection to remove unwanted particles such as dust, but to keep all the active components.

PROPOLIS ANALYSED

Analysts have gone to great lengths to try to discover what it is about propolis that is so exceptional. The material is made up of 50 to 55 per cent resins and balsams, 30 per cent beeswax, 10 to 15 per cent essential oils and 5 per cent pollen.

It was when the analysts started looking more closely at the micro-components that a clear picture began to emerge. The most active part of propolis seems to be the compounds termed flavonoids that are present in the resins collected from the trees. It is the flavonoids that have such remarkable properties in controlling micro-organisms and stimulating the immune system in humans. It is worth looking at these effects in considerably more detail.

Chapter 12

PROPOLIS — FIGHTING DISEASE AND PROMOTING HEALTH

'Adapt the remedy to the disease.' — Chinese proverb.

Propolis is believed to fight disease in two ways. It stimulates the immune system, which is the body's natural defence mechanism, and it either kills or severely incapacitates infectious organisms such as bacteria, fungi, and viruses.

Professor Chavin, who has carried out a great deal of work in Paris on the disease-fighting aspects of propolis, says that the material will increase the body's immunity to colds, flu, coughs, tonsillitis and cystitis.

A NOTE OF CAUTION

A few people are sensitive to propolis and tests at the Edinburgh Royal Infirmary showed that in Britain approximately one person in every 2000 might show a puffy redness of the skin when it has been touched by propolis. Some beekeepers are sensitive to propolis, which must be quite a problem as they continually come into contact with it, but a silicone barrier cream has been shown to be effective. Also, it does not seem to lessen the good effects of propolis when taken internally or as a gargle.

The way to safely test for sensitivity is to rub a little of the propolis product on the side of the nose. If it quickly goes very red, then you are the one in every 2000 that should avoid propolis. Test again from time to time as sensitivities do change.

BOOSTING THE IMMUNE SYSTEM

Work carried out by Drs Balalykin and Orkin showed that propolis actually stimulates the cells in the body that destroy invading organisms. These cells, known as phagocytes, literally engulf unwanted invaders and destroy them. Dr Orkin injected mice with propolis after they had been exposed to a bacterial infection. He found that after a few hours the mice which had received propolis had more than twice as many phagocytes fighting the infection as the animals which had received no propolis.

Professor Havsteen of Kiel University explains that propolis is also effective in stopping viruses getting into cells and causing illness. Our bodies are constantly bombarded with all sorts of minute infective organisms and our immune systems succeeds in fighting off a great many of them. A virus only gets a hold if it manages to penetrate the fortifications of the body's tissues and force the cells to manufacture thousands of identical units of the virus. One person catches a cold or flu and then manufactures a large supply of additional infective organisms that are subsequently breathed, coughed or sneezed over everyone else. The illness is prevented if the body can keep the virus out of its cells. Professor Havsteen believes that this is how propolis works.

A virus particle will try to trick the body's cells into removing its outer coat and thus expose its nasty infective part. If the immune system is under par the body will be fooled by this ploy and will do as the virus says and take off its overcoat. Once removed, the virus shows its true colours and invades the cell, forcing it to make the army of future viruses. Professor Havsteen believes that the flavonoids in propolis actually prevent the body from taking off the virus's overcoat.

Professor Kuhnau of Hamburg University believes that flavonoids, such as those in propolis, should be a regular part of our diet in order to stimulate the immune system against its daily dose of potentially harmful microbes. Furthermore, the antioxidant activity of flavonoids acts to prevent cell damage and improve the absorption of certain nutrients.

Professor Osmanagic put these theoretical findings to a practical test when a particularly virulent epidemic of influenza was sweeping through his native town of Sarajevo. He chose a group of people who were in particular danger of succumbing to the infection because of their close contact — a training college where nursing students and teachers were working together during the day but returning to their homes in various parts of the town in the evenings.

Students and teachers who were without any symptoms of influenza at the time were invited to take a teaspoonful of Melbrosin propolis diluted with honey every day for between forty and fifty days. It turned out that some of them could not be bothered and so in the end 63 from six classes took the product and 157 did not.

Only about one in ten of the students who took propolis became infected and half of those caught their flu only three or four days after beginning the preventive treatment so there would have been very little chance of their resistance building up. Those who decided not to take the propolis fared extremely badly in comparison. Almost one in four of them succumbed to the infection, compared with one in ten of those taking the preparation. The teachers who took propolis did even better; only one in twenty-five was ill, and then only mildly. The lack of illness among the teachers taking propolis was especially valuable as so many of their colleagues (those not taking propolis) were off sick, leaving the college short staffed.

KILLING BACTERIAL AND FUNGAL INFECTIONS

Not only will propolis help to prevent microbes from infecting the body, but it also kills or incapacitates the microbes themselves. Microbiologists study the effects of a particular material in the following manner. They prepare sterile dishes of a savoury jelly which are kept covered at all times to prevent infection from particles in the air. They then apply minute amounts of microbes to areas on the jelly and leave them to grow at the required temperature. Many microbes multiply at frightening speeds; for example, one type doubles its quantity in twenty minutes. If there are 20 microbes at the start, there will be 40 after twenty minutes, 80 after forty minutes and 1,280 after two hours. When the microbiologists wish to study the effects of an antibiotic they add the required amount to the dish and check the growth of the microbe in its presence.

One of the first studies on the antibiotic effect of propolis was carried out in 1960 in Russia by Dr Rabinovic. In his experiment Dr Rabinovic collected some of the infective organisms from patients suffering from tuberculosis. He allowed these organisms to multiply under carefully controlled conditions and then looked at the effect of propolis on their subsequent growth. He demon-strated that propolis stopped the multiplication, and thus had the ability to prevent the spread of the disease.

Three years later Dr Kivalkina looked at the growth of other bacteria, and found propolis to be effective against several, including one causing sore throats (Streptococcus aureus). Perhaps the most comprehensive study on the effects of propolis on the growth of microbes was carried out in 1967 by Dr Lindenfelser. Not only did Dr Lindenfelser look at 39 types of bacteria, 39 types of fungi and two yeasts, but he also looked at 15 different types of propolis collected from different areas of the USA. He then proceeded to apply the propolis in different concentrations to find out how much was needed to kill the microbes.

Lindenfelser demonstrated that propolis is very effective in preventing the multiplication of 25 of the 39 species of bacteria and 20 of the 39 species of fungi. The two yeasts were particularly resistant to the effects of propolis. Some of the 15 samples of propolis were more effective than others, depending on the type and quantity of flavonoids collected by the bees from the trees.

Professor Havsteen believes that propolis is superior to antibiotics such as tetracycline, penicillin, and streptomycin. These three are harvested from micro-organisms, whereas the flavonoids of propolis come from trees, which are much more advanced in terms of evolution. Professor Havsteen suggests that the human body is much more able to tolerate treatment with propolis than with antibiotics which cause the suppression of some essential reactions in the body. Professor Havsteen points out that the presence of antibiotics produced from microbes may alert the body's defences which recognize the components as coming from organisms generally considered to be foreign. The fact that medical progress has made the antibiotics 'friendly' isn't necessarily recognized by the body's immune system which may proceed to attack the foreign material. Many people are allergic to penicillin and there are a number of other reactions which can occur which must be considered detrimental to the progress of curing the illness in question.

ENHANCING ESTABLISHED ANTIBIOTICS

In addition to being an antibiotic in its own right, propolis can enhance the effect of other antibiotics. Drs Kivalkina and Gorsunova carried out experiments where they looked at the effects of known antibiotics with and without added propolis. They made sure that the quantity of propolis was not, in itself, sufficient to prevent the multiplication of the microbes.

Their results showed that small quantities of propolis strengthen the effects of the antibiotics tetracycline, neomycin and polymycin. The strength of these antibiotics was increased between ten and one hundred-fold by the presence of propolis when used on one particular type of bacterium ('gold shimmering staphylococcus'). The strength of the antibiotics streptomycin, penicillin, neomycin, polymycin, and tetracycline was increased by a similar amount in the presence of small quantities of propolis, when applied to cultures of coliform bacteria. The presence of propolis in these small quantities does not stop the microbes from becoming resistant to the antibiotics.

Propolis is also useful in extending the effective life of antibiotic salves. Without propolis a salve containing a standard antibiotic will have a shelf life of two to three months. When propolis is added the shelf life increases to between nine and twelve months, a quite remarkable improvement.

ANTIOXIDANT ACTIVITY

In 1922 a Hungarian scientist, Dr Albert Szent-Gyorgi, discovered vitamin C. Ten years later he discovered that vitamin C cures scurvy. He found out that the vitamin encourages the repair of the tiny blood capillaries that break during scurvy, and that vitamin C prevents the disease in the first place. His main sources of vitamin C were citrus fruits and paprika, and he busily extracted the life-enhancing nutrient. He soon discovered something else. He found another nutrient that apparently boosted the power of vitamin C. He showed that this new nutrient also helped maintain healthy capillaries and he chose to call it vitamin P. Today we call it something else. We use the term *flavonoids*.

The flavonoids in propolis are valuable in keeping the capillaries in peak condition, and they also help to boost the power of vitamin C by preventing its oxidation and working with it on the blood vessels.

The flavonoids are one of the class of antioxidants, whose importance to health is becoming clearer day by day. The antioxidants maintain the integrity of cells by trapping free radicals that can otherwise cause damage and hasten the ageing process. The flavonoids also possess the ability to bind heavy metals such as lead, mercury, and cadmium, to prevent these from causing damage to the body.

REDUCING TOXICITY

Some unpleasant diseases are characterized by the production of toxins which, by definition, are poisonous to the body. One such disease is diphtheria. This illness is caused by a microbe called *Corynebacterium diphtheriae* which not only produces a ghastly fever, pain and difficulty in breathing, but releases toxins which cause inflammation of the heart muscles and additional pain. Thankfully, these days diphtheria is preventable through vaccination.

Dr Karimova and his colleagues at the Kasan Medical Institute looked at the effects of propolis on the toxin produced by the diphtheria bacterium. He discovered that propolis is protective against the effects of the toxin. His experiments were carried out on guinea pigs and showed that those given a dose of diphtheria toxin and propolis did not show the characteristic effects of intoxication and local cell damage. In comparison, the poor animals that did not receive the propolis actually died of the effects of exactly the same amount of administered toxin. These animals were not able to enjoy the protective effects of propolis.

ENHANCING VACCINATION RESULTS

The process of vaccination against a specific disease involves introducing a safe form of the illness into the body which stimulates the immune system to make a supply of antidote. Once this antidote has been manufactured by the body it remains available for a considerable time (sometimes for life) and fights off any subsequent attack by the real disease.

Dr Balaykina wanted to see whether propolis would improve the immune response to disease organisms. He prepared safe extracts of the food poisoning microbe called *Salmonella enteritidis* (a common parasite of rodents). He then immunized rabbits and mice with the preparation and kept checking them to monitor the animals' response. As expected, their immune system went to work and produced antibodies to fight off any subsequent attacks by similar organisms. Dr Balaykina then injected a similar number of animals with a mixture of the same preparation from the food poisoning microbe, together with a measure of propolis.

The results of the study showed that the animals receiving propolis produced a faster and better immune response to the disease challenge than shown by the control animals. In other words, the propolis actually stimulated the animals' natural disease-fighting abilities.

OTHER APPLICATIONS

It is said that Stradivarius, the most famous violin maker the world has ever known, insisted that propolis be included in the varnish on his creations. Perhaps this was one of the factors in perfecting the unsurpassed tone?

The healing powers of propolis can be incorporated into massage oil. A good recipe is 5 grams of propolis to 100 millilitres of a good carrier oil such as coconut oil. Mix these two well (using a blender if available). If you wish to try a different version occasionally, try adding three or four drops of essential oil of lavender at the end. The lavender not only adds a pleasant aroma, but has a calming effect and is similar to propolis as it is an antioxidant and is used to ease rheumatism.

There is one particular area of research into propolis that demands considerably more study. Drs Popovici and Oita in Romania carried out investigations into the effects of propolis on cell division. They looked at cells from the common onion and added a substance that causes the nuclei of the cells to divide unnaturally quickly. They then added a weak solution of propolis at the same time as the cell division agent, and observed that the nuclei did not divide. Thrilled with their findings, these researchers put forward the suggestion that propolis might just have some application in the future in the treatment of cancer cells, which, of course, divide unnaturally fast. If in years to come this is proven, then propolis may be claimed to have yet another healing application. At this point in time it is far, far too early to make any such statement.

Dr Gonnet of France has also looked into the effects of propolis on plant cell division. He showed that propolis tends to slow down the growth of otherwise healthy lettuce seedlings. The common link between the two studies is that both used cells whose role is to grow quickly. Much more research is needed here before any conclusions about cancer may be drawn. All we know at this stage is that propolis is harmless to animal cells, but it does have the ability to slow down the division of certain plant cells.

It seems likely that the ability of propolis to inhibit cell division is a clever way of ensuring that pollen in the beehive does not germinate. After the process of flower pollination the particle of pollen undergoes cell division to enable it to grow down towards the female reproductive organs. Propolis can act to inhibit this growth, thus stopping pollen in the beehive bursting into active growth.

Chapter 13

PROPOLIS TO EASE PAIN AND INFLAMMATION

'Sweet is pleasure after pain.' — Dryden 1697

Propolis is useful to the human body in a wide variety of ways. In this chapter we will concentrate on its beneficial effects in easing pain, reducing inflammation and allergic responses, and as a mild anaesthetic.

MODE OF ACTION

Professor Havsteen of Kiel University believes that propolis acts to reduce pain in a manner similar to aspirin. He states that propolis is a pain-killer derived from natural and not synthetic sources and is unlikely to cause any of the side-effects that are associated with aspirin itself. The Professor believes that propolis, like aspirin, stops the body producing prostaglandins in response to an infection or physical damage. In this instance the pain, inflammation, and fever are caused by the release of prostaglandins, and if these can be reduced the symptoms will disappear. In common with so many of the other actions of propolis, it is believed that the flavonoids are the components that are active in reducing pain.

A similar explanation is offered by Professor Havsteen when considering the development of an allergic response to an irritant. In the case of an allergic response the swelling, redness and itching are caused, not by prostaglandins, but by a substance called histamine. As soon as the body detects an irritant the immune system leaps into action and attacks the invader. The fighting troops muster at the battle site, whether it be an insect bite or hay fever irritating the mucous membranes of the nose. Histamine is released by special fighting cells called mast cells, and this compound stimulates the attack on the invader. An allergic response causes a great deal of unnecessary misery for the sufferer and the discomfort can be reduced by something that gets rid of the histamine (often called an antihistamine). Professor Havsteen suggests that the flavonoids in propolis act to stop the release of histamine by the mast cells. He likens it to the effect of propolis on virus particles, where the immune cells refuse to agree to take off the outer coat of the virus so it is unable to release its active centre. In the case of an allergic response, the particle causing the problem (the allergen) tries to get the mast cell to form an extremely close relationship so it can transfer its nasty message into the heart of the mast cell. The next step would be the release of histamine, but the flavonoids act to prevent the relationship from getting too close in the first place, so the histamine is never released.

People who suffer from allergies generally find they get a reaction to many different stimuli. Pollen itself can be used prior to the hay fever season in order to confer immunity. Without immunity, pollen can continue to cause problems with hay fever sufferers. If you are the type of person who suffers from hay fever, and you wish to take advantage of the beneficial actions of propolis, you must make sure that the propolis you use is free from pollen particles, unless you have already gone to the trouble of developing an immunity to pollen prior to the hay fever season.

ANAESTHETIC EFFECT

In addition to easing pain, propolis acts as a local anaesthetic. The combination of the two is extremely helpful in many situations, for instance, for sore throats or the treatment of ulcers. But propolis can be used as an anaesthetic in its own right, as shown in a study carried out in Bulgaria by Dr Tsakoff.

Dr Tsakoff used sheep and dogs, giving them both local and general anaesthetics. He used a solution of propolis in dilute alcohol and compared this to the effects of the anaesthetic novocaine.

He carried out minor incisions on the animals and concluded that the propolis preparation was just as effective as the preparation of the standard anaesthetic, novocaine. Dr Tsakoff did note that some of the sheep developed an area of swelling where the propolis solution had been applied locally. This swelling developed after 24 hours, and took a further two to three days to subside. The dogs showed no such reaction. This study indicates that propolis can be used as an effective anaesthetic.

SORE THROATS

It was in June 1967 that 'Mr Propolis' (K. Lund Aagaard) first discovered the benefits of propolis in treating sore throats. Mr Propolis had to attend a function even though he had been suffering from a bad sore throat for a few days. In the evening his temperature rose to 40°C and his throat was so sore and swollen that he was unable to eat a meal. In desperation he turned to the propolis he had been collecting for years.

He crushed a little of the dried propolis with a pestle and mortar and dissolved the powder with some warm water. He then filtered the mixture through a coffee filter to produce a yellow liquid that looked a bit like a weak cup of tea. During the evening he gargled with the liquid two or three times, and just before he went to bed he drank the rest of the potion. To his absolute astonishment, in the morning Mr Propolis found himself in excellent health. His swollen throat had returned to normal, and the soreness had reduced to a small red spot instead of the raging inflammation of the previous day. He concluded that propolis must contain strong antibiotic and anti-inflammatory components to exert such a dramatic effect in just a few hours. How right he was.

Needless to say, Mr Propolis was very excited about his discovery and lost no time in telling all his friends and acquaintances. His interest in the effects of propolis spread like wildfire to include studies on 16,000 people throughout Scandinavia between 1967 and 1973. At one point he voiced his concern when he discovered that a few people are actually allergic to propolis and he looked more closely at this problem. In a detailed study of 1,700 people using propolis, only three of them showed an allergic response.

His studies showed propolis to be effective in the treatment of 97 per cent of the patients, with only 3 per cent showing no improvement.

Although propolis is known to be an effective treatment for sore throats, it is also extremely good for other disorders of the mouth, nose, and ears. It is worth looking at a few medical trials and case histories in order to appreciate the full value of this extraordinary material.

INFLAMMATION OF THE TONGUE

Doctors call this painful condition glossodynia. It can have a number of different causes, including infection with the increasingly common Candida albicans, or infection with other microbes due to a decrease in the quantity of the body's natural antibiotic or in the acidity of the digestive juices of the stomach. The body's natural antibiotic is called lysozyme, and it is normally present on the surface of the skin and on the moist membranes of the nose and mouth. Lysozyme is an important part of the immune system, an enzyme that kills off invading microbes.

A study carried out in Romania by Dr Muresan looked at the effect of propolis on 50 patients suffering from inflamed tongues. The causes of the disorder were varied, as recorded above, but the common fact was that they had all been given a variety of drugs that had been unsuccessful in curing the problem. The ineffective drugs included antibiotics, anti-fungal preparations, and cortico-steroids. The propolis was administered as a mouthwash for 10-30 days.

The study was carried out as a double-blind trial so that half the patients were given a mouthwash that contained no propolis, nor anything else that could possibly effect a cure. This was to make sure that the study checked the action of the propolis itself and not the action of using a mouthwash or even the effect of a little tender loving care.

The results showed that the propolis treatment brought an improvement in 56 per cent of the cases. It brought a complete cure to one third of the patients, with no return of the disorder in subsequent months. A further quarter of the patients felt a great deal better for the treatment although their tongues did not heal properly in the 30 days of study. The remaining patients showed no improvement, but it should be remembered that these people's mouths were full of microbes that had repeatedly resisted all previous forms of medical treatment. The fact that propolis helped so many patients after such a long time is remarkable.

INFECTED GUMS AND MOUTH

The healing, regenerative, and anaesthetic powers of propolis form an ideal combination in the treatment of painful conditions of the mouth and teeth. Dental decay (caries) can destroy so much of a tooth that the sensitive central soft pulp starts to complain bitterly (a condition known as pulpitis). Hot and cold foods cause distress to the patient and chewing becomes virtually impossible. The bacteria that produce the acid that eats into the teeth can also cause painful inflammation of the gums.

Research in Russia, Czechoslovakia, and Germany has repeatedly shown that propolis helps in the treatment of dental and mouth disorders in three ways. The direct application of a propolis solution with alcohol serves to anaesthetize the painful tooth prior to commencing the appropriate dental treatment. After the treatment propolis acts to reduce the bacterial population that would otherwise exacerbate the inflammation and potentiate the infection. Finally, propolis aids in the regeneration of healthy tissue so the mouth can heal fully. This last attribute is extremely helpful after the extraction of a tooth. The flavonoids are effective in repairing damaged capillaries (as Dr Szent-Gyorgi discovered over 50 years ago) and it is the flavonoids in propolis that help repair the gum tissue after the extraction.

Scientific reports in the use of propolis to treat painful teeth include studies by Drs Marcenko, Mitinia, and Davydova. These researchers treated 130 patients (85 five women and 45 men) suffering from toothache. During the treatment they applied a paste made with propolis dissolved in alcohol and mixed with zinc oxide. At the end of the study the efficacy of the propolis paste was measured by subjective comments and by tapping the teeth to see whether they were still painful. The results showed a definite improvement in 99 (three-quarters) of the patients, 11 individuals showed a small improvement, and the remaining 20 continued to suffer. In order to establish why a small proportion of the patients did not respond to propolis treatment, the researchers looked at X-rays taken at the start and the end of the study. They discovered that even before the trial, the non-responders were showing a spread of the inflammation from the pulp inside the tooth to the area of gum surrounding the tooth. In conclusion they recommended that propolis is suitable for the treatment of inflammation of the centre of the tooth, provided the disease has not advanced so far that the surrounding gum tissue has become infected. In the latter case it may be necessary to remove the damaged tooth prior to successfully treating the cavity with propolis.

PAINFUL, INFLAMED CONDITIONS

Propolis also goes to work on inflammation of the muscles and joints. A series of studies carried out in Austria investigated the effect of a cream containing propolis on patients complaining of a wide variety of painful conditions. The cream, *Melbrosia Propolis Salve*, contains pine resin and larch resin in addition to propolis.

Drs Eckl and Dworak, from Ruette, carried out a double-blind medical trial on 56 patients. As in all double-blind trials, the researchers were given two products that looked identical. One was active propolis salve, the other was and inactive or placebo ointment. Most of the patients were in hospital for the treatment of illnesses such as heart disease or breathing disorders, but additionally they were all suffering from painful joints or muscles. This study concentrated entirely on the effects of the two ointments on the painful joints or muscles. Of the 56 patients, 27 were suffering from arthritis, 18 from lumbago or other back pain, 8 from muscular pain (myalgia) and 3 from painful elbows. The treatment consisted of massage of the affected area several times during the day and the application of a film of cream and dressing over night.

The results showed that 28 (precisely half) of the patients receiving the propolis ointment showed an 'impressive improvement' after a few days of treatment (between two and seven days). Only 4 individuals showed a similar improvement after treatment with the inactive, placebo ointment.

The two doctors were particularly impressed by the way the patients showed no adverse reaction to the propolis treatment. They commented that the drugs normally used in the treatment of rheumatism tend to produce unpleasant side-effects, particularly in elderly patients. The doctors showed that the propolis salve is highly acceptable and commended its use. They concluded that *Melbrosia Propolis Salve* offers 'a fast and clear reduction of pain; easing of morning stiffness and peripheral joint ailments and is easily tolerated'.

SPORTS INJURIES

Between April and August 1984 the Institute for Sports Medicine at the Bosnian town of Sarajevo, Yugoslavia, treated 112 injuries with propolis salve. Almost half of the injuries occurred on the soccer pitch, with the other half coming from basketball, handball, and athletics, with minor contributions from karate, volleyball, and boxing. The injured were all within the age range 17 to 25, with a 77 per cent to 23 per cent ratio of males to females. Over half the injuries were bruises, one quarter joint sprains and the remainder swellings.

The study was carried out by Drs Nedazad Brkic and Ismet Arlanagic, who pointed out that sportsmen and women are always keen to overcome the pain of their injuries in order to be able to get back to training and competition as soon as possible. Pain is the feature that tends to stop participation, rather than disability due to the injury itself.

The participants were seen as soon as possible after being injured, either on the same day or the following morning. After the diagnosis, each patient was treated by massaging a small quantity of propolis salve over the affected area. In a few cases the damaged area was covered with a dressing. Thereafter, further applications of propolis salve were given over a period of two to five days. The total number of treatments varied between four and ten.

The patients noticed the pain-killing effect of the propolis preparation as soon as one hour after application. On the second day they noticed a reduction in inflammation. After three days, three-quarters of the patients reported that the pain had disappeared completely, and the majority of the sportsmen and women were able to resume training and competing after five to seven days of treatment.

In this particular study the organizers did not arrange a double-blind trial where the treatment is tested against an inactive placebo. However, the Sarajevo Institute of Sports Medicine has an excellent reputation for the treatment of sports injuries and their doctors are experts in this specialized area. Drs Brkic and Arslanagic carried out a careful study of the effects of the propolis salve and concluded that it offers 'important qualities for the alleviation of pain and for the prevention of secondary infections of injuries, so we can recommend it as a really excellent remedy for the treatment of acute sports injuries'.

Chapter 14

PROPOLIS TO HELP HEAL

'There is a remedy for everything could men find it.' — Herbert
1640.

In addition to fighting disease, and easing pain and inflammation, propolis acts to promote healing. It is particularly valuable
in the treatment of burns, ulcers, and skin disorders. It is also
useful in the treatment of post-operative ear infections and breathing difficulties in children. Perhaps the area that shows the greatest
potential is the ability of propolis to counteract the devastating
effects of Candida albicans, which is spreading so rapidly.

BURNS
For years, Russian and Romanian doctors have treated burns with
a propolis spray. The spray contains alcohol as well but this quickly
evaporates to leave a fine film of propolis on the surface of the
burn. The propolis acts to ease the pain, reduce the inflammation, fight off invading micro-organisms and help the healing
process.

  Dr E. Muresan and his colleagues in Romania carried out a study
where he compared the healing of burns dressed with propolis
and burns treated with an ointment made with penicillin and sul-
phathiasol. In each case the treatment was given daily Dr Muresan noticed that after 24 hours the burns treated with propolis
were dry and the local swelling was decreasing. In comparison
the burns treated with the medicated ointment still looked wet
and the surrounding tissue was swollen. After six days the propolis-
treated burns were progressing nicely; they were covered with a

fine dry crust and showed no symptoms of infection. At this time the burns receiving the ointment treatment were covered with a thick crust under which the tissue was still swollen and showing considerable infection from micro-organisms. After twelve days the propolis-treated burns looked good, with skin forming well, minimal scarring and no hard tissue. It took a good 20-24 days before the other treatment produced healing tissue, and even then there was considerable scar tissue with irregular thickened areas.

Dr Muresan concluded that the propolis spray worked extremely well in the treatment of burns. He did add that he felt the propolis should be used in the form of a spray rather than in an ointment, as the latter would tend to prevent the burn from drying adequately during the healing process. We should like to add that if you have to treat a burn yourself, the recommended first aid treatment is to cool the damaged tissue as soon as possible. For example, a burned finger should be plunged into cold water without delay. The cooling process restricts the damage to surrounding tissue. When the area has cooled, you should then allow it to dry before dressing it.

ULCERS

Propolis has been used with considerable success in the treatment of stomach and duodenal ulcers. Dr A.G. Gorbateno looked at 126 patients in the Reproval Hospital in Perejaslaw-Chmelnizkij over a period of six years. The patients were mainly men over 50, more than half of whom were suffering from the severe, active form of the illness.

Their treatment consisted of taking propolis in quarter of a glass of milk, one-and-a-half hours before eating, three times a day. The propolis was taken as a 30 per cent solution in alcohol and 50-60 drops of this mixture were added to each glass. Some patients were unable to tolerate milk so they took water instead. All the patients were given a suitable diet and the regimen was continued for between 21 and 28 days. X-ray examinations were carried out before the treatment, after seven days and three months after the end of the treatment.

Although the majority of patients had been suffering from their ulcers for between three and five years, the propolis cured the pains of three-quarters of all the subjects within three to four days. The characteristic problem of unwanted muscle tension in the front part of the stomach wall did not subside for another three to four days. The patients' heartburn, nausea and vomiting stopped almost at the same time as the pain disappeared. Dr Gorbateno particularly noted the fact that propolis had a biostimulating effect on the patients, beginning with an improvement of general condition and continuing with the normalization of sleep, the lessening of irritability and an increase in cheerfulness.

The efficacy of the treatment with propolis depended on the length of the illness prior to hospitalization. It proved least effective with those patients who had been ill for more than ten years prior to the study. One of the best ways to establish the efficacy of a treatment for ulcers is to see whether the troubles return months or years after the initial treatment. This study showed that over three-quarters of the patients stabilized so well after propolis treatment that they were still free of problems after five years. There were thus considered completely cured. By comparison, other studies using more conventional medicines showed almost half the patients complained of the return of their problems within the first year after treatment.

The propolis treatment was not completely successful for a number of patients: 6 per cent of them had an allergy to propolis and thus had to receive other medicines instead. A further 16 per cent showed a relapse of their condition some time after the initial treatment, but their ulcers responded once more to propolis. The doctors discovered that most of the relapses had been caused by excessive physical exertion.

Dr Gorbateno and his colleagues concluded that propolis is a good treatment for ulcers, pointing out that propolis promotes a faster recovery than treatment with other common medicines. He also referred to the fact that propolis normalizes the production of acids in the stomach.

Propolis has also been used successfully for getting rid of troublesome and irritating mouth ulcers. A little dab of propolis tincture, containing between 2 and 5 per cent of propolis, for two or three days generally cures them completely. This treatment is suitable for children.

SKIN DISORDERS

Propolis has been used successfully in the treatment of a wide number of skin problems, including acne, itching, childhood eczema, shingles (Herpes zoster) and warts and verrucae. Propolis, applied either in the form of ointment or solution (tincture), acts to combat the infection as well as promote healing.

In cases of bad acne or other nasty spots a tiny dab of propolis tincture every day (preferably several times a day) will promote rapid healing. The propolis will reduce the local inflammation so the redness subsides, as well as forming an invisible protective coat on the blemish. The healing effect of propolis produces healthy skin growth after the spot has disappeared.

Drs T.V. Vinogradova and G.P. Zajceva achieved particularly promising results using propolis in the treatment of children infected with microbial eczema and suffering from itching skin. Other doctors have shown that propolis is effective in eliminating itching with other causes, although they achieved no success with nettle rash or acute eczema.

Shingles, or Herpes zoster as it is medically termed, is painful and unpleasant. At a symposium on api-therapy in Portoroz, Yugoslavia, Dr Franz Feiks talked of his experiences in using propolis in the Klosterneuburg Hospital in Austria. He explained how he had treated the local skin sores of shingles with a 5 per cent solution of Melbrosin propolis tincture, applying the solution daily. In the 21 cases he treated, the pain disappeared in two days and did not reappear. In 3 of the cases itching persisted for a long period of time, while in all others this common accompaniment to shingles disappeared. Indeed, in 19 of the patients the skin sores were healed without any recurrence and only 2 cases had a subsequent development of their illness.

Warts and verrucae tend to be particularly resistant to the treatments suggested by many doctors. A favourite treatment is the regular application of formaldehyde which is a poison that destroys all the skin in the area. This dead skin is then scraped off, hopefully together with the offending wart or verruca. A daily or twice daily application of propolis tincture is a good and safe alternative, and seems to work much more quickly and more effectively.

EAR INFECTIONS

The ability of propolis to kill micro-organisms has been shown to be valuable in promoting healing in the middle ear. Drs I.A. Kurilin and T.E. Samraj tested 100 patients who had developed complications after ear surgery. Prior to the treatment they removed samples of the pus in the ear and analysed this to discover the type of microbes present. They discovered a whole host of microbes that are resistant to antibiotics such as penicillin, streptomycin, and tetracycline. It was hardly surprising that the infections were not healing with conventional treatment. To the delight of both the researchers and the patients, the microbes were found to be sensitive to propolis which quickly killed off the infection.

The treatment consisted of removing the pus from the ear, cleaning the surfaces with a dilute solution of alcohol and then placing a loose dressing covered with a 33 per cent propolis salve in the cavity. The doctors found that after six to nine days the microbes has been completely killed off and the area was free of germs. Complete recovery was enjoyed by 62 of the patients after the propolis treatment, but a further 27 showed only a temporary recovery as some of the microbes returned after a couple of months, and 5 per cent of the patients showed an allergic response to propolis.

BREATHING DIFFICULTIES

Research in Kiev has shown that propolis is beneficial in the treatment of children suffering from the difficulties in breathing associated with bronchial pneumonia and bronchial asthma. The children's treatment consisted of spraying the affected area with a fine mist of propolis in dilute alcohol. The spray treatment was carried out between five and twenty times. Dr Tanasienko, who carried out the research, showed that in the majority of cases the improvement was marked and infections subsided.

Drs Skalozub and Melnilova carried out further studies at the

Donezk Medical Institute and found the most favourable results in children suffering from pneumonia accompanied by asthmatic components. They showed that after three or four inhalations of propolis spray the patients' coughing lessened and in due course disappeared altogether. After five to six days of treatment the condition of the lungs had improved enormously.

CANDIDA ALBICANS

The fungus Candida albicans is assuming plague proportions; in fact in Germany the situation is reported to be getting worse every day. Every other person is said to suffer from some kind of chronic fungus infection. Such parasites invade the skin and hair, eat the beds of the nails, and inflame the lining of the lungs and even the inner walls of the heart. Our living habits and our civilization have made possible the spread of this mini-relation of the mushroom.

Fungus can only survive where it is warm and damp, for example in nylon socks and rubber boots, under nylon petticoats, in central heating, and in the fluffy fur of pet animals. Hygiene and the use of drugs has also worked to the advantage of the fungus. Every anti-bacterial substance gives the fungus more room to move. In fact, the very use of antibiotics can suppress the bacteria which would normally keep the fungus in check.

Candida is a particular problem because it grows everywhere in hospitals: in the air, on the floor, and even on the nurses themselves. They often don't notice it because they have a strong resilient constitution but there is certainly a danger to patients weakened by operations and through the administration of drugs.

Statistically speaking, in Germany every third vagina is infected with Candida albicans. Some doctors blame the pill and a very free sex-life among the young. The hormones in the pill change the constituents of the secretions in the vagina increasing the proportion of glycogen creating an environment very suitable for the spread of fungus.

It now looks as if work with propolis will provide the remedy. A propolis pessary is achieving remarkable cure rates. Scientific work to prove this began with a group of four doctors led by Dr

Ishida of the Tohoku University School of Medicine in Japan.

This work was carried on by Dr Cizmarik and Dr Troupl, of the University of Bratislavia, who tested propolis on a whole range of fungi and achieved a high standard of results. They extended their trial in 1976 and concluded that propolis is a substance with remarkable effectiveness for all fungal infections of the skin and body.

PROPOLIS — PRACTICAL USE

All the signs are that propolis, while not being any sort of cure-all, simply has to be in every first aid box, medicine cabinet, hospital pharmacy, and doctor's bag. As more products become available, so the range of the field of applications becomes greater.

Preparations which it is useful to include in your first aid box are a propolis salve, tablets, capsules, and a tincture (5 per cent propolis in alcohol). Tinctures are produced by a number of manufacturers, and may be taken as drops on a (raw) sugar cube or mixed with a drink. Products which have been particularly recommended are:

Melbrosin propolis salve This is a special massage cream which is effective in treating aches, sprains, and sports injuries.

Ortis propolis and bran tablets These contain 50mg of propolis in each tablet.

Reevecrest garlic and propolis capsules Again with 50mg of propolis per capsule.

Food Supplement Company propolis tincture Available in bottles containing 14ml.

Chapter 15

ROYAL JELLY

There's food for gods! There's nectar! There's ambrosium!' —
Shakespeare, *Julius Caesar.*

Royal jelly has been a source of interest and intrigue for centuries. To this day we still do not know exactly how this elixir stimulates the human body, but we do know that thousands of people swear by its properties and take it daily to produce improved health and a sense of well-being.

In the hive, royal jelly is a truly exceptional food. It is this magic material that turns an ordinary worker bee into a magnificent, fertile queen. There is no doubt that it contains all the nutrients necessary for this amazing transformation; nutrients that are essential to the human as well as to the bee. It is a superfood, a substance that can turn the ordinary into the extraordinary.

A number of scientists have tried to investigate the properties of royal jelly, but much of its magic remains a mystery. Most of the scientific research into royal jelly has been carried out in Russia and eastern Europe, but the studies are limited in number in comparison with those on pollen and propolis.

NATURAL SUPERFOOD

A beehive houses between forty and sixty thousand worker bees. Each one of these has special glands at the side of her head which secrete droplets of royal jelly. This is a milky-white light textured jelly that to us tastes slightly sharp. This royal jelly is the food of all the bee larvae in their first three days of life — it gives them a vital boost of nutrients to set them up for an exceptionally busy future.

When the bee larvae emerge from their eggs there is no difference between the worker bees and potential queen. The other bees, the drones, are different because they hatch from unfertilized eggs. The newly hatched workers weigh 0.15 milligrams. After three days the worker selected to become queen goes on getting royal jelly as her daily superfood, whereas the workers turn to a mixture of honey, pollen and water. After the first five days the queen's weight has increased a staggering two thousand fold. Her sisters, the workers, weigh only half as much.

The queen reaches her full size extremely rapidly and after a mere 16 days she is sexually mature. In comparison it takes the workers 21 days to reach maturity, and even then they remain small and sterile. The queen is ready to start laying eggs 16 days after hatching from the egg, and she sets out to lay up to two thousand eggs every day for the rest of her life. These two thousand eggs are equivalent in weight to her own body weight, and royal jelly is the food that enables her to be so fecund. Not only is this a staggering achievement in itself, but the queen goes on to live for between four and five years. Her sisters, the workers, live for only 45 days in the height of the summer season.

ANALYSIS
Royal jelly has been scientifically analysed and found to contain:

	percentage
water	66
carbohydrates	14
protein	13
fat	5

The remaining 2 per cent contains a wealth of vitamins, minerals, some hormonal activity, a natural disinfectant, and a supply of the agents acetylcholine and inositol.

The carbohydrates in royal jelly are all natural sugars such as glucose, fructose and sucrose. The protein is rich in all the amino acids essential to life and has an abundance of the other amino acids that the body would otherwise have to manufacture itself. All the components of the protein are present in a fine and unique balance that is just right for promoting growth and development without waste. And the fat content is low, in keeping with today's recommendations on good nutrition.

Royal jelly is especially rich in the B vitamins. It has a good supply of the group required for releasing energy from food into the body. These vitamins are B1 (thiamine), B2 (riboflavin), niacin, pantothenic acid, and biotin. It also contains vitamin B6 (pyridoxine) which is essential for the metabolism of proteins and is considered an anti-stress vitamin, and folic acid and vitamin B12. These last two are required to prevent anaemia. All are vitally important to the body, and if they were absent from the diet the body would not be able to obtain its energy, nor would it be able to maintain healthy blood.

Although royal jelly is an excellent source of the essential B vitamins it is not a good source of the vitamins A, C, D, and E. Vitamins A, D, and E are soluble in fat, not water like the B vitamins, and tend to be associated with foods rich in oil like wheatgerm oil and fish liver oil. Vitamin C is found in citrus fruits and many fresh fruits and vegetables. Bees do not need vitamin C so it is not in their food. Oddly enough, humans and guinea pigs are the only animals to require regular vitamin C, and we must turn to other sources to obtain sufficient supplies of this vitamin.

Minerals and trace elements such as calcium, copper, iron, phosphorus, potassium, silicon, and sulphur are represented in royal jelly. It is also rich in acetylcholine (1 milligram per gram of royal jelly) which is an essential ingredient for the correct transmission of nerve impulses in humans. Another component is the compound inositol which acts in a variety of ways in the human body. Inositol helps to remove fats deposited in the liver and acts to reduce the amount of cholesterol in the blood. It is also known to be a mild anti-anxiety agent and is associated with the maintenance of a healthy head of hair.

Finally, royal jelly contains a natural disinfectant. It is believed that this is present in order to destroy any microbes that might try to attack the developing bee larvae while they are inert and dependent on royal jelly as their food.

DEVELOPMENT AND SEXUALITY

We know that worker bees are unable to reproduce, whereas the queen bee must be one of the most fertile of all living organisms. Apparently the only thing that determines whether a young bee larva will become a worker or a queen is whether a youngster is fed royal jelly every day or just at the start of her life. If this seems too much like a fairy tale I can assure you that it has been proven again and again. If the queen dies or leaves the hive, the workers will instantly start feeding up another perfectly ordinary worker bee larva to become the next queen. In fact this process is utilized in the production of royal jelly on a commercial scale; the queen is removed and lots of worker bee larvae, less than 36 hours old, are introduced into the hive in a specially prepared frame of hygienically prepared cells. The adult workers respond immediately by making a large quantity of extra royal jelly to feed the potential queens.

There is no doubt that royal jelly is the miraculous substance that enables the queen to develop ovaries and become supremely fertile, as well as growing at a rate that is twice as fast as the workers. But does the formula work for other animals? As usual, it is very difficult to test the hypothesis on humans, unless a pair of identical twins agreed at birth to be subject to a detailed scientific study for the next 20 years of their lives. One would receive royal jelly and the other would not and their growth rate and sexual development could be monitored closely. Clearly this would be a preposterous and impossible experiment, but the work has been carried out on some of our smaller distant relatives, ones that grow and develop quickly enough to monitor.

In 1977, a group of research scientists (A. Salama, H. H. Mogawer and M. El-Tohamy) from the Egyptian National Research Centre in Cairo looked at the growth of baby female rats with and without royal jelly. The rats weighed an average of 37 grams to start with and were given royal jelly in addition to their food. After four weeks the rats that had been given 40 milligrams of fresh royal jelly every day had increased their weight to 79 grams. Those that had been given a dummy dose of 0.5 millilitres of water and no royal jelly had only reached 60 grams by the same time.

The researchers looked at sexual development as well as rate of growth. At the beginning of the third week of the study, each female rat was transferred to the bedroom of a virile male. In the morning each female was removed from her male and put back into her own cage for the day. The nightly visits continued until the end of the fourth week, the time when the expectant mothers were left alone to contemplate the arrival of their first brood.

As soon as the babies were born the researchers worked out the date on which conception occurred. The earlier the date, the earlier the female had reached sexual maturity and had become fertile. The results showed that the females receiving 40 milligrams of royal jelly every day reached sexual maturity after an average of 26 days. By comparison, those who had no royal jelly did not reach sexual maturity for a further 16 days, over half the time again. These results clearly show the incredible potency of royal jelly.

The Egyptian scientists also compared the action of fresh royal jelly with freeze-dried (lyophilized) royal jelly preparations. Those receiving the freeze-dried version grew faster and matured earlier than the rats that had no royal jelly, but the results were not as good as with the fresh royal jelly. The freeze-dried royal jelly rats grew to 71 grams in comparison with the fresh royal jelly rats' 79 grams. Furthermore, the freeze-dried preparation brought the rats to sexual maturity after 30 days, compared to 26 with fresh royal jelly. The researchers draw attention to the extra potency of the fresh royal jelly in comparison to the freeze-dried preparation.

ROYAL JELLY AS A TONIC

Many people take royal jelly as a general tonic and pick-me-up. It is difficult to discover exactly how the substance acts within the human body, but studies with animals have provided a few clues. Research scientists Peichev and Uzbekova have shown independently that brain, heart and liver tissue take up more oxygen after royal jelly has been administered. This means that these tissues have somehow been stimulated to become more energetic and to work harder. The animals that did not receive any royal jelly showed no such effect.

Some researchers suggest that royal jelly may act as a type of hormonal stimulant, a bit like the stimulant adrenaline. It is really too early to draw valid conclusions in this area, but it has been proved that royal jelly contains some hormonal activity. The researchers J. Vittek and B.L. Slomiany have been successful in isolating a compound which appears to be identical to the steroid hormone testosterone which is active in vertebrates.

Studies carried out in Bulgaria by Dr P. Peichev suggest that royal jelly can be particularly beneficial to the elderly. Dr Peichev has observed that subjects receiving royal jelly show an improved general state with better nervous control. Much of Dr Peichev's work relates to the wide variety of beneficial effects of taking a royal jelly and honey mixture and it is therefore a little difficult to interpret which material has which effect.

ROYAL JELLY AS AN ADAPTOGEN

Royal jelly is considered to be an adaptogen, that is, a natural substance that acts in the human body to increase resistance to harmful chemical and biological occurrences. A true adaptogen has to act to normalize whatever process has gone wrong, for example, an adaptogen should raise blood pressure that is too low or lower blood pressure that is too high.

The scientific literature is peppered with tantalizing snippets of information about the wide variety of actions that have been observed after taking royal jelly. In addition to the scientific studies there are thousands of people who have purchased royal jelly and have themselves experienced some of the advantages of this extraordinary material.

It is widely believed that royal jelly exerts a beneficial action on both the composition and the pressure of the blood (scientific studies have been carried out independently in these areas by Drs Lupachev, Beslekoev and Mishchenko). From his studies in New York, Dr Young T. Cho reports that a number of patients taking royal jelly showed a lowered blood cholesterol count as well as an improved sense of well-being.

Royal jelly has been used beneficially in the treatment of bronchial asthma and angina pectoris (Drs Kogut and Bogacheva). There has even been a report from Canada (Drs Townshend and Morgan) to show that royal jelly afforded protection to mice against artificially prepared cancer cells. No one should draw the conclusion that these results might be applicable to humans, but it provides us with something to think about. There is also subjective evidence that royal jelly is beneficial in the treatment of allergies and asthma.

One day scientists may find the key to unlock the mysteries of royal jelly so we may discover exactly how it works inside us. At the moment all we can say for certain is that is has been shown to have a wide range of beneficial actions; as a food, a tonic, an agent to induce a sense of well-being and as an adaptogen. One thing is certain: it is not necessary to wait for the scientists to tell us royal jelly is beneficial to health. That has been proved already.

Chapter 16

WHICH BEE PRODUCT?

'Remedies do cure without a Physician, but not a Physician without remedies.' — Robert Wittie 1651

Bee preparations are formulated in a number of different ways and from many sorts of flower. The different manufacturers have concentrated on different aspects of the virtues of pollen as well as propolis and royal jelly but all have found that there is a considerable overlap so that it is a matter of individual trial and error to find which is best for you and your particular need — all will be good but some will be outstanding.

This chapter, then, is to give you some useful guidelines concerning products that have been tried and tested. There are other good makes available in different parts of the world but most of the types available are described here. Let us begin with the simplest and most natural pollen.

ORTIS

Adolf Horn founded the company Ortis in a nature park of unpolluted open countryside in the highest part of Belgium. From the very first the keynote of Ortis, which is now run by his two sons Michel and Philippe and his widow Irene, has been quality. For example, so that they could be sure that ginseng, which they mix with royal jelly to form a valuable elixir, was of the required quality, they did not just use powder which may not be as good as the exporter pretends it to be, but ground the whole roots themselves. This made the product really work and it was found that the royal jelly potentiated the effects. This product is called *Ginseng Royal*

Jelly and Vitamin E. They produce *Royal Jelly in Solution* and *Royal Jelly Capsules; La Gelée Royale* and *Honey Royale* are also excellent products. Good for the skin and for healing eczema is a royal jelly cream called *Creme Royale.* Ortis produce pollen granules from pesticide-free bee traps which brush the pollen from the legs of the bees as they go into the hive, and also tablets containing propolis and bran which are very good for mild infections and sore throats.

However, the supreme Ortis royal jelly product is *Api-Fresh.* This contains four easy to open vials which contain nothing but fresh unadulterated raw royal jelly which, like all their royal jelly products, is flown in specially from China where a very high standard of production is scientifically controlled. *Api-Fresh* has been recommended by many experts including Leslie Kenton. It is delivered in insulated containers by first class post, either to the retailer or, in case of difficulty, direct to the consumer.
The addresses of Ortis are, in Belgium:
  Ortis SPRL
  B 4740 Elsenborn
  Belgium
and in the UK:
  Ortis (UK)
  PO Box 223A
  Thames Ditton
  Surrey KT7 0LY

MELBROSIN
Paul Urban, a great Austrian patriot, founded Melbrosin many years ago when he found how effective certain bee products were. His company has been at the forefront of carrying out clinical tests on pollen products and these include studies on the menopause, failing libido, slowing down the ageing process, protecting patients undergoing radiotherapy, and in sport.

Melbrosia for Men is made from the fermented 'bee bread' or perga which is painstakingly removed by skilled workers from the honeycombs where it has been subjected to a natural process of fermentation. This is combined with ginseng and royal jelly and has been found very effective. (Table 1 in the Appendix shows the composition of bee bread.)

For women there is *Melbrosia PLD* (which stands for 'pour les dames') which is a mixture of different pollens to that used in the product for men, together with royal jelly and vitamin C. This has had extensive clinical trials and is especially valuable for the older woman.

Melbrosia Propolis Salve is a useful addition to the first aid box and is a unique massage cream which is almost miraculous in its quick and positive effect on such trying home and sporting afflictions as tennis elbow, housemaids knee, and all sorts of muscular aches and sprains. Trials with ballet dancers and footballers have shown that the propolis salve can mean that performances can take place that would otherwise require substitutes.

For internal use, a 5 per cent tincture of propolis in alcohol is effective; prepared by several manufacturers, including Melbrosin, it can be taken on a raw sugar lump or in a drink.

The addresses of Melbrosin are:

Melbrosin International
Vienna A11915
PO Box 185
Austria

and in the UK:

c/o Reevecrest
The Old Mill
Godalming
Surrey GU7 1EY

REGINA

The founder of Regina, Irene Stein, has been extremely successful in making people aware of the advantages of royal jelly. She launched the company in 1974 and has since made a successful share issue on the unlisted market.

Her book *Royal Jelly* is a best seller and she has spoken much about the virtues of her products on radio and television.

They include *Royal Jelly Capsules, Regina Royal 5, Royal Concorde, Royal Jelly and Vitamin E Cream* and *Regina Royal 100.*

The address is:
  Regina Royal Jelly Limited
  Regina House
  2-3 Elstree Gate
  Elstree Way
  Boreham Wood
  Herts WD6 1JD

WASSEN

Ray Matthews, the founder of Wassen, was the first to make the British public aware of the health benefits to be derived from pollen. He set himself a daunting task because one of the problems with pollen is that the outer coat of the grains is so tough that a lot has to be taken in order for a good effect to be felt.

He developed a technique for micronizing the pollen and stabilizing it by natural means so that small tablets were very effective. His product is called *Pollen-B* or, in America, *Bee Pollen from England*.

Pollen-B is generally the most convenient and effective way of taking a pollen supplement, either as a general health insurance or as a treatment.

The address is:
  Wassen International Limited
  14 The Mole Business Park
  Leatherhead
  Surrey KT22 7BA

REEVECREST

Apart from representing Melbrosin in the UK, Reevecrest's founder, Bernd Linke, leads a very innovative team.

An effective and useful product, good for sore throats and mild infections, is the *Reevecrest Garlic* and *Propolis Capsules* which contain 50mg of propolis per capsule.

Useful products from other companies include the 14ml propolis tincture from the Food Supplement Company of Godalming.

Healthcrafts, major suppliers of nutritional products, include in their extensive range three different strengths of royal jelly capsules and and an excellent *Premiere Fresh Royal Jelly* which comes on boxes containing ten phials which you just open and drink. The address of Healthcrafts is:

Booker Nutritional Products Limited
Beaver House
York Close
York Road
Byfleet
Surrey KT14 7HN.

SOME USERS REPORT

Scientific reports are fundamental to the understanding of pollen therapy, but it is good to read the actual words of some of those who have found that pollen and other bee products really work for them and for their families.

General health and vitality

Mrs M.M., Clacton-on-Sea
I find Pollen-B tablets excellent and all that is said of them is quite true. I am 68 years old and have more energy and less aches and pains than I have had for years. I must thank you for that most sincerely.

Mrs D.J., Peckham
I wish to compliment you on *Pollitabs*. My husband, three children and myself have taken a course of these remarkable tablets and the result has been incredible! After only a few weeks I can actually notice a stunning difference in the children and my husband — they are much more energetic and lively. Thank you very much indeed.

Mr. J.W., Weybridge
My wife and I have been taking *Pollen-B* for approximately three months now and have found it beneficial to our health and general well-being. As we are both in late middle age this assistance to our energy problem is most welcome, and I would thoroughly

recommend *Pollen-B* to people of all ages for whom the question of coping with the strains and stresses of our modern way of life is of paramount importance.

Mrs T.S., Walton-on-Thames
Melbrosia PLD capsules are worth their weight in gold. I was having a very rough time in life and in desperation tried *Melbrosia* and after just one month's treatment I simply could not believe that I was the same person. My tranquillity was restored, fears dispersed and I am now beginning to look much younger.

Convalescence
Mrs A.H., London
In the first place I was given *Pollen-B* by mistake at the chemist's shop so I thought I would try them out. I have now been using them for three years and since taking them I felt much better, having had heart surgery in the past. The doctors at the hospital said I now have the blood pressure of a young girl, my age being 62.

Mrs C.B., Dunstable
I was recovering depressingly slowly following a 'woman's operation' when a friend recommended *Melbrosia PLD*. I simply had to write to tell you how much better I am. I had almost forgotten what it was like to feel in good health but now I do believe that I am even better than before.

Mr J.L., Leeds
To climb to the very top of Ilkley Moor, all the steps to the top of York Minster and up all the steps to my flat on the fifteenth floor are things that have been done by others. So what is so special about this? Well! three months ago I had a coronary, my second in two years, thus leaving me with angina.

A bit dispirited, with people telling me 'Oh! you have had it now.' People tell me to take it easy, I suppose they meant well. But I have taken *Pollen-B* tablets and with determination I have done all the things I mentioned. I intend to keep on taking them and do really think there must be something very special about them.

Mr L.L., Johannesburg

I was given a bottle of *Melbrosia* in order to help me regain my health after a very severe operation and a long period of recuperation.

I am already feeling infinitely better and would like you to arrange to send me six or more bottles as soon as you can.

Nerves

Mr P.S., Gallway

Thank you for *Pollen-B*

I suffered from nervous tension, doctors were no good with their modern cures. I got back my health, my energy, my personality from *Pollen-B*. Once again thank you.

Mr M.E., Newbury

Just over eighteen months ago I had a nervous breakdown and was beginning to feel I would never be able to manage without tranquillizers. Having reached the stage where I would try almost anything I bought a six months supply of *Pollen-B*. After taking them for a month I found I was able to go without tranquillizers and the length of time has now stretched to almost three months. I wouldn't be without *Pollen-B* for anything now.

Mrs R.T., Perth

I was beginning to get, so my husband tells me, absolutely impossible to live with (I'm at the time of the 'change') when the assistant in the health store recommended that I took *Melbrosia PLD*. I must say that I did not really believe in it and I thought that I was wasting rather a lot of money but the transformation was nothing short of a miracle. Your product has turned what was for me proving to be a very difficult time of life into a truly happy experience with no problems. My nerves and my temperament are back to normal. Perhaps you have saved a marriage!

Prostate troubles

Mr S.B., Glasgow

I feel I ought to write to tell you how I have been saved from having an operation which my doctors said was quite essential. I was having very serious trouble with the prostate gland (I am 75) and all arrangements were made for me to go into hospital when a great friend who only believes in herbal treatment said that if he had known he would have got me to try pollen which he was sure would have done me good. Anyhow I thought it was never too late to try anything and went immediately to the herbalist and bought some *Pollitabs*. Within two days my trouble had disappeared and the following day I had to go to the hospital to have some photographs taken. These showed absolutely no trace of any of my trouble and all the difficulties with my water have ceased. Now they say that I do not need an operation.

J.B., London
I have just returned from abroad and I am completely out of *Cernilton* (strong *Pollitabs*). It is really quite marvellous and — so far — has kept surgery at bay for an enlarged prostate. I did not believe that anything could do the job and had never even heard of the product. But it works!

Dr H.T., Vienna
I write to tell you about a patient who is one of my family who has experienced a wonderful return to health with three *Florapoll* (Melbrosia) capsules each day. This 89-year-old has suffered from a long time from a continual enlargement of the prostate. So much so that he has to carry a catheter. He has also had a long standing infection of the urinary tract. This has been resistant to antibiotics and sulpha drugs. Then we used *Florapoll* with the intention of helping the prostate and not only was that improved but we also found that the infection was cured also. This meant that we were able to stop the ineffective treatment with antibiotics and can report that even now the tract is remaining in good condition.

Mr C.J., Long Beach
My daughter from England sent me a six-month's supply of *Pollen-B* to correct prostate troubles. After using it I got excellent results in reducing the prostate gland and also what I did not expect — increased virility and that is what I wanted all the time.

Virility and rejuvenation

Mrs M.S., Cowes

I have been a regular user of *Pollen-B* for six weeks and feel years younger. I passed through the change of life some twelve years ago, but all the old excitement is returning. This is very puzzling. I definitely put it down to the rejuvenating effect of *Pollen-B*.

Dr J.B., Scotland

For the past three years my sex life was a bit troubled and I was having great difficulty. But since being on *Melbrosia for Men* I have returned to normal. All in all, I find them very good and definitely feel more relaxed in my everyday routine.

Breasts

It has often been noted that pollen improves muscle tone and very many women have reported that this has resulted, for them, in an enlargement and firming of the breasts.

Miss R.O., Enfield

I am a housekeeper working in a stately home and in the course of my duties meet many important and interesting people. I have always had extremely small breasts which have been a source of acute embarrassment to me even though friends often tell me that people take no notice of such things. Perhaps I was a little silly about it but there was nothing I could do.

I then tried a course of *Melbrosia PLD* because of what I have read and the results have been wonderful. My breasts have gained two inches in size and altogether they are firmer and better shaped. Also I feel much better and more relaxed in myself. I am writing in the hope that my experience can help others.

Miss M.B., Malta

I am very pleased with the effect of *Pollen-B*. My eyes are brighter and my hair is more beautiful. My breasts are firmer and the pimples I had on my face are nearly all gone. These effects came after only one month. I am taking two tablets a day, one first thing in the morning and the other last thing at night. I thank you very much for all you have done.

Allergies

Mr J.J., Buckhurst Hill

I feel I must write to say how well I have felt after taking *Pollen-B* for over a year.

I usually suffer from bronchial asthma but did not even have a cold this winter.

Mrs C.B., Darlington

I have been taking *Pollen-B* for just over a year and I thought that you might be interested to know that I am delighted with the results. After four weeks all hard and rough skin had gone from my heels and legs and now after a year the tone and condition of all my skin has improved. My hair has thickened and improved in texture. I have had asthma for many years and whether it is due to the tablets I really don't know but the breathlessness and wheezy attacks which I had, have now become less frequent. I feel much better and I also sleep better.

Mrs M.H., Malaga

Melbrosia PLD completely cured my rough and patchy skin. When I stop taking it I am as crotchity as an old bear, with all sorts of menstrual pains etc., but when I take it I feel wonderful.

Mrs S.J., Israel

I have always suffered from a very dry skin with eczema and scaling and since taking a course of *Melbrosia PLD* as a tonic to my amazement the skin has improved beyond all recognition.

Mr N.R., Totnes

My doctor said that it would be unwise of me to take a course of *Pollitabs* because I suffer from hay fever and I am very allergic to pollen. I went ahead anyway and he said he would keep his eye on me. You will be glad to know that not only has *Pollitabs* made me feel a lot better than I have felt for years. I also had less hay fever than I can ever remember having even though the pollen count was unusually high.

Gastric problems

Mr J.H., Penzance

I write to tell you that the tablets my doctor gave me which I need for another condition make me constipated and that since taking *Pollen-B* I have been helped considerably. Thank you.

Miss C.P., Barton

I would like to say that since taking *Pollen-B* I have never felt better. I always used to suffer from an upset stomach and a lack of appetite. Now I can eat a full meal and feel no uneasiness at all after it. I cannot praise them highly enough.

Mr T.S., Suffolk

For two years now every time I have been feeling unwell for whatever reason I have taken a course of *Melbrosia*. I have been delighted with how often it has done the trick for me. I take it when I am constipated and I take it when things go the other way but the effect always seems to be the same — I return to normality. When in your life you have been as ill as I have you can have no idea how wonderful it is just to feel normal.

Migraine

Mr J.K., Stroud

I started taking *Pollen-B* tablets last July. Since then they have had a marked effect of my general health. For years I have suffered from migraine headaches and I have tried every known form of medication including making several visits to the Migraine Clinic at St Bartholomew's Hospital in London. In the nine months that I have been taking the tablets the headaches are becoming less and less. Coupled with this I am less tense and this has had unexpected side-effects, such as not being dependent upon laxatives which I had taken regularly for years. I now go for long periods without needing to have recourse to them. It is marvellous after years of suffering to be free of the pain and bad migraines, also the necessity for constantly taking analgesics.

Hair and nails

Mr R.W., Cheshire

It is now over nine months since I first started a course of *Pollen-B*. The benefits that have accrued from this are now really too numerous to mention. Suffice to say that at the age of 64 I have regained the energy that I had when I was 40 — I have been completely bald for over twenty years and now I have a covering of hair all over the bald part — I have recommended pollen to hundreds of friends and in no single case has there been anything but praise.

Mrs T.S., Southall

I was advised to take *Melbrosia PLD* to help me because I often suffer from painful periodic pains. I am glad to tell you that these have been lessened but, even more remarkable, my brittle nails and lustreless hair are problems of the past! It has taken almost a year but now, for the first time, I really do have a 'crowning glory'.

Mrs A.R., Aylesbury

I think that *Pollen-B* is fantastic. My nails have actually grown properly for the first time for years, I am energetic and I look younger than I ever did.

One thing bothers me and I hope that you will advise me about it. I am on a contraceptive pill and wonder if this would affect *Pollen-B* in any way. I sincerely hope not as I would not want to stop taking my daily pollen. I would rather give up the pill.

(*Note:* Pollen has not so far been reported as being incompatible with any medicament or with the pill, so she is quite safe to go on using both.)

Colds

Mrs T.N., Birmingham

I write as the mother of a large family (six — four boys, two girls). They all travel to school on buses and, for years, we have suffered with colds they have caught on the way to school and at school. I am writing to tell you about the wonderful results we have now achieved by using two of your products. This is what we do. For the last two years, at the beginning of autumn we have all (mum and dad too) taken a 30 day course of *Melbrosia* pollen and then, as soon as people start to catch colds around us we take propolis capsules. This has meant that during these last two years none of the family has caught a bad cold. When someone does start a slight sniff he or she is immediately given one gram of natural vitamin C every three hours. At the same time we all take more propolis and pollen! It is not apparently a cheap way of doing things with eight people in the family but I am sure that the treatment has paid for itself because none of us have had a day off work or school now for two years whereas before, between us, a total of two months away in a year was not uncommon. By the way, the children all seem brighter too and we have not caught any of the other diseases such as flu even though there was one serious epidemic in our neighbourhood.

Mr R.B., Adelaide
My son who is a travelling musician in Australia has found *Pollen-B* tablets most beneficial. He says he has not had a cold whereas all the others around him have and he swears he does not get as tired even after all the long late hours of work.

Mr P.P., Rotherham
I work in a crowded office and caught every cold that was going so regularly that I felt embarrassed in case my colleagues thought that I might be malingering.

I was recommended to try a course of *Pollitabs* throughout the winter and now I am writing to you to say that even though on one occasion there were only 3 of us left out of 25 all the others being down with colds and flu, I was able to work harder than ever before, and felt fine.

Diabetes
Mrs J.B., Stockport
My young son who has diabetes has recently discovered *Pollen-B*. He has been taking them for a couple of months and he has

felt very much better since taking them. He had been in and out of hospital and could not sleep very well and was getting worse and worse. He is now much more relaxed and sleeping well again. Before taking the tablets he had to go to the clinic every six weeks but now he only goes every six months.

Mr R.F., Richmond
I am only a mild diabetic but the complaint does seem to have left me very tired and listless. I thought I would try a course of *Pollen-B* and now I have noticed a change in myself and do not get as tired and exhausted as I used to.

Among the many other letters which are not included are ones concerning the very good effect of *Melbrosia* on the periodic difficulties of adolescent girls where 50 girls out of 60 with serious problems in a boarding school (enough to prevent them working) were cured; reports of help for colitis sufferers; relief of giddy spells and the confusion of the elderly.

Another book could be written from the hundreds of letters praising the virtues of pollen. It is hoped that the selection given in this chapter will abundantly illustrate the importance of the scientists' findings in human terms. For it is people, their health and happiness — what is often called the quality of life — that we must aim to improve in this modern and perhaps too technologically minded world.

The work which began with Greeks like Herodotus in 400 B.C., with Celsus and then Dioscorides in the first century A.D.; as well as that mentioned in the Koran and in Persian and Arabic manuscripts of the sixth and eighth centuries which mention propolis for the treatment of eczemas, for blood purification and for bronchial catarrh; all these things have been part of the developing picture of medicine throughout these thousands of years. We now have the technology and expertise to test them thoroughly and make them available to all mankind.

Pollen, honey itself, bee bread, royal jelly and propolis: these golden gifts to man are in true worth beyond price and yet can be made accessible even to the humblest peasant. As the great Frenchman, Voltaire, said in 1755: 'Nature is inexhaustible'.

Controlled trial proves the power of pollen

The *Farming Today* programme on BBC Radio 4 in the early hours of 21 December 1988 featured the writer Montague Keen, who presented the first news in Britain of the soon-to-be-published research findings of Professor El Hamdi of Egypt.

The occasion was the International Apiculture conference in Cairo.

The professor wanted to discover, using tests on humans and laboratory animals, whether honey, the magic elixir used from the times of the Pharaohs and still renowned folk medicine in Egypt, was as good as legend told.

The first trial was to confirm a use described elsewhere in this book: honey for the healing of open wounds. Three methods were used to treat wounds of equal size: a saline treatment, *Savlon* antiseptic, or an application of honey. The clear result was that honey was far quicker as a healer than the two orthodox treatments and also, unlike those, there was no scarring of the tissues.

Next, the Professor tried an extraordinary and much harsher test and that was for the patients to take the honey by mouth instead of putting it on the wound. This worked even better!

Then he took a group of 20 pregnant women who were suffering from the common condition that many pregnant women find inconvenient and unsightly: oedema, which is a general swelling caused by the retention of fluid in the tissues. This is often coupled with high blood pressure and a high level of uric acid. He gave them a tablespoonful of honey three times a day for a week, after which 15 of the 20 were completely cured.

The Professor wondered why all were not cured and so he checked where the honey had come from and found that the 5 who were not better had used honey made in the winter from bees which had been fed on sugar, and not the natural honey full of pollen which the bees gather from flowers. He added pollen to the honey and made sure that it was all mixed up and then every single one of the patients was cured.

Obviously, more work needs to be done on finding which flowers produce the best results and, indeed, whether the honey is at all necessary in this particular case. The Professor is continuing his work but meanwhile we must be sure to see that the honey we use at table is not the filtered heat-treated sort from which all vital nutrients are excluded, but the real stuff, pollen and all.

This is yet another example of a way that simple, safe, traditional medicinal techniques can be given necessary support through sympathetic modern scientific evaluation. It is not 'rational' to say that small quantities of nutrients present in pollen or in royal jelly or in other products of the bee can have a curative effect except for bees; but the fact is that there is much more to discover of what it is that brings such remarkable successes from the beehive. So good luck to Professor El Hamdi and to other pioneering scientists who will one day find the scientific answers to healing processes which are not yet understood. Meanwhile, take advantage of the work that has been done and enjoy the benefits for yourself and your family.

APPENDIX

TABLE 1
The composition of pollen and bee bread (g per 100g material).

	Pollen	Bee Bread
Water	24.3	23.8
Protein	24.1	23.3
Sugars	22.8	30.4
Starch	1.8	0.0
Fat	4.9	5.4
Fibre	9.3	11.1
Non-combustible matter	3.2	2.8

TABLE 2
Amino acids present in pollen samples

	Zea mays 1954	Alnus glutinosa	Pinus montana
Amino acids	+	+	+
Alanine	+	−	−
α-Amino-butyric acid	+	+	+
Arginine	+	+	+
Aspartic acid	+	+	+
Cystine	+	+	+
Glutamic acid	+	+	+
Glycine	+	+	+
Histidine	+	−	−
Hydrocyproline	+	+	+
Isoleucine	+	+	+
Leucine	+	+	+
Lysine	+	+	+
Methionine	+	+	+
Phenylalanine	+	+	+
Proline	+	+	+
Serine	+	+	+
Threonine	+	+	+
Tryptophan	+	+	+
Tyrosine	+	+	+
Valine	+	+	+

TABLE 3

Amino acid content of pollen samples (g of amino acid per 100g protein)

	Zea mays 1953	Zea mays 1954	Alnus glutinosa	Alnus incana	Pinus montana
Arginine	6.3	5.7	9.8	6.2	6.4
Leucine	7.6	5.6	6.0	7.1	6.5
Lysine	5.9	5.0	4.7	5.0	5.1
Methionine	1.6	1.6	1.4	1.6	1.5
Phenylalanine	2.9	2.3	2.3	3.0	2.1
Tryptophan	0.6	0.6	0.8	0.4	0.8
Tyrosine	1.9	1.9	1.7	1.9	2.1

TABLE 4

Vitamins in pollen samples (μg/g pollen dry weight)

	Zea mays 1953	Zea mays 1954	Alnus glutinosa	Alnus incana	Pinus montana
Riboflavin	5.7	6.2	11.2	12.1	5.6
Nicotinic acid	40.7	71.8	82.7	82.3	79.8
Pantothenic acid	14.2	12.7	4.2	5.0	7.8
Pyridoxine	5.9	5.5	5.7	6.8	3.1
Biotin	0.52	0.55	0.65	0.69	0.62
Inositol (mg/g)	30	30	3.0	3.5	9.0
Folic acid	2.2	2.2	0.53	0.64	0.42

TABLE 5
The fats present in pollen samples (g per 100g extracted fat)

Saturated fats:

Caprylic	0.1
Capric	0.6
Lauric	0.9
Myristic	0.2
Palmitic	26.5
Stearic	4.1
Arachidic	3.2
Behenic	1.8
Lignoceric	0.3

Unsaturated fats:

Oleic	15.8
Linoleic	26.2
Linolenic	18.7

Ratio of unsaturated fat to saturated fat 1.6 to 1.0

Minerals present in pollen:

Calcium	Silicon	Chlorine
Phosphorus	Sulphur	Boron
Iron	Sodium	Molybdenum
Copper	Selenium	
Potassium	Titanium	
Magnesium	Zinc	
Manganese	Iodine	

INDEX